Hands-on guide to
clinical pharmacology

CHRISTOPHER TOFIELD
General Practice Registrar
Waikato District
New Zealand

ALEXANDER MILSON
Senior House Officer (Surgery)
Bristol Royal Infirmary
Bristol
United Kingdom

SUKHDEV CHATU
Senior House Officer (Medicine)
Queen Elizabeth Hospital
London
United Kingdom

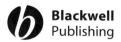
Blackwell
Publishing

© 2005 C. Tofield, A. Milson, S. Chatu
Published by Blackwell Publishing Ltd
Blackwell Publishing, Inc., 350 Main Street, Malden,
  Massachusetts 02148-5020, USA
Blackwell Publishing Ltd, 9600 Garsington Road, Oxford
  OX4 2DQ , UK
Blackwell Publishing Asia Pty Ltd, 550 Swanston Street,
  Carlton, Victoria 3053, Australia

First published 2000
Reprinted 2001, 2002, 2004
Second edition 2005

Library of Congress Cataloging-in-Publication Data

Tofield, Christopher.
  Hands-on guide to clinical pharmacology / Christopher Tofield, Alexander
Milson, Sukhdev Chatu.—2nd ed.
    p. ; cm.
  Chatu's name appears first on the earlier edition.
  Includes bibliographical references and index.
  ISBN 1-4051-2015-0
  1. Clinical pharmacology—Handbooks, manuals, etc.
  [DNLM: 1. Drug Theraphy—methods—Handbooks. 2. Pharmacology,
Clinical—methods—Handbooks. QV 39 T644h 2005] I. Milson, Alexander.
II. Chatu, Sukhdev. III. Title.

  RM301.28.C48 2005
  615′.1—dc22

                                                                    2004021822

A catalogue record for this title is available from the British Library

Set in 8.5/10pt by Kolam Information Services Pvt. Ltd,
Pondicherry, India
Printed and bound in India by Replika Press Pvt. Ltd

Commissioning Editor: Vicki Noyes
Development Editor: Nicola Ulyatt
Production Controller: Kate Charman

For further information on Blackwell Publishing, visit our website: http://
www.blackwellpublishing.com

The publisher's policy is to use permanent paper from mills that operate a
sustainable forestry policy, and which has been manufactured from pulp
processed using acid-free and elementary chlorine-free practices.
Furthermore, the publisher ensures that the text paper and cover board used
have met acceptable environmental accreditation standards.

Contents

Preface

The first edition of *Hands-on Guide to Clinical Pharmacology* was written whilst we were medical students at St Bartholomew's & The Royal London Hospital School of Medicine and Dentistry. At that time, we were in need of a practical yet concise set of notes to revise clinical pharmacology. What had initially been a collated set of revision notes was expanded upon, structured and turned into the first edition of this book. Some time has passed since then and, with research in pharmacology marching on, it became evident that an update was needed.

In this second edition, we have presented information on 127 drugs, which you are most likely to encounter on hospital wards or during your course of study. Sections containing both treatment regimens of common conditions and detailed information on the relevant drugs will help the reader obtain a better understanding of therapeutic management.

This book has a twofold purpose:
1 To provide a study aid for all students involved in the study of clinical pharmacology.
2 To serve as a user-friendly reference on the wards.

It has been designed as a learning tool and is not intended to provide an exhaustive account of clinical pharmacology. We have selected important interactions, adverse effects and contraindications as are relevant to students. Doses have purposely been omitted (with a few important exceptions) since these are not relevant to students and are best obtained from a local formulary. For a full list of interactions, adverse effects, contraindications and drug doses, the *British National Formulary* or other appropriate formulary should be consulted.

Whilst aiming to ensure accuracy of the text, we have at the same time attempted to maintain conciseness – a feature that is much valued by students. Those memories of impending exams with stacks of thick textbooks to read have not been forgotten!

We hope this book will help you come to grips with pharmacology in a clinical setting and, above all, take the stress out of pharmacology exams.

C. Tofield
A. Milson
S. Chatu

Acknowledgements

Getting the first edition of *Hands-on Guide to Clinical Pharmacology* off the ground was a laborious undertaking, especially since at the time we were final year medical students at St Bartholomew's & the Royal London Hospital School of Medicine and Dentistry. We have particularly fond memories of our two pharmacology professors, who not only lent us a helping hand with the first edition of this book but also guided the medical students heroically through the weeks and days running up to pharmacology finals.

We thank Professor Nigel Benjamin for his unfailing support and Professor Mark Caulfield for his inspiration and sound advice.

We gratefully acknowledge the following for their helpful suggestions toward this edition:

Dr M. Behan, Specialist Registrar in Cardiology

Dr G. Coakley, Consultant in Rheumatology

Dr J. Collier, Consultant in Psychiatry

Dr E. Gamble, Consultant in Respiratory Medicine

Dr C. Gibbs, Consultant in Endocrinology

Dr E. Hamlin, Consultant in Neurology

Dr S. P. K. Linter, Consultant in Intensive Care

Dr C. Mansell, Clinical Microbiologist

Dr S. Metcalf, Consultant in A&E Medicine

Dr A. Perez de Velasco, Specialist Registrar in Dermatology

Dr C. Probert, Consultant in Gastroenterology

Dr C. Shakespeare, Consultant in Cardiology

Mr V. P. Singh, Consultant in Obstetrics and Gynaecology and Reproductive Medicine

Dr A. P. Whaley, Consultant in Intensive Care

Abbreviations

ABG	Arterial blood gas
ACE	Angiotensin-converting enzyme
ADH	Antidiuretic hormone
ADP	Adenosine diphosphate
AF	Atrial fibrillation
ALT	Alanine transaminase
AMP	Adenosine monophosphate
APTT	Activated partial thromboplastin time
5-ASA	5-aminosalicylic acid
AST	Aspartate transaminase
ATP	Adenosine triphosphate
AV	Atrioventricular
BCG	Bacillus Calmette–Guérin
BMI	Body mass index
BP	Blood pressure
BPH	Benign prostatic hyperplasia
CBT	Cognitive–behavioural therapy
CCU	Coronary care unit
cGMP	Cyclic guanosine monophosphate
CHD	Coronary heart disease
CMV	Cytomegalovirus
CNS	Central nervous system
COC	Combined oral contraceptive
COMT	Catechyl-O-methyl transferase
COPD	Chronic obstructive pulmonary disease
COX	Cyclo-oxygenase
CPR	Cardiopulmonary resuscitation
CSF	Cerebrospinal fluid
CT	Computerised tomography
CTG	Cardiotocography
CVA	Cerebrovascular accident
CXR	Chest X-ray
D.C.	direct current
DMARD	Disease-modifying antirheumatic drug
DNA	Deoxyribonucleic acid
DT	Diphtheria, tetanus
DTP	Diphtheria, tetanus, pertussis
EBV	Epstein–Barr virus
ECG	Electrocardiogram

ECT	Electroconvulsive therapy
FBC	Full blood count
FEV	Forced expiratory volume
FSH	Follicle-stimulating hormone
GA	General anaesthesia
GABA	Gamma-aminobutyric acid
GI	Gastrointestinal
GP	General Practitioner
GTN	Glyceryl trinitrate
HAART	Highly active antiretroviral therapy
Hb	Haemoglobin
HBsAg	Hepatitis B surface antigen
HDL	High density lipoprotein
Hib	Haemophilus influenzae type b
HIV	Human immunodeficiency virus
HMG CoA	3-hydroxy 3-methylglutaryl co-enzyme A
HOCM	Hypertrophic obstructive cardiomyopathy
HRT	Hormone replacement therapy
5-HT	5-hydroxytryptamine
Ig	Immunoglobulin
IHD	Ischaemic heart disease
IM	Intramuscular
INR	International normalized ratio
ISA	Intrinsic sympathomimetic activity
ISDN	Isosorbide dinitrate
ISMN	Isosorbide mononitrate
ITU	Intensive therapy unit
IUCD	Intrauterine contraceptive device
IV	Intravenous
LABA	Long-acting beta 2 agonist
LDL	Low-density lipoprotein
LFT	Liver function test
LV	Left ventricular
LVF	Left ventricular failure
MAO	Monoamine oxidase
MAOI	Monoamine oxidase inhibitor
MI	Myocardial infarction
MMR	Measles, mumps, rubella
MRSA	Methicillin-resistant *Staphylococcus aureus*
NMDA	*N*-methyl-D-aspartate
NRTI	Nucleoside reverse transcriptase inhibitor
NSAID	Non-steroidal anti-inflammatory drug
PCA	Patient-controlled analgesia
PCI	Percutaneous coronary intervention
PDE_5	Phosphodiesterase type 5
PE	Pulmonary embolism

PEF	Peak expiratory flow
PID	Pelvic inflammatory disease
POP	Progestogen-only pill
PUVA	Psoralen with ultraviolet A
RNA	Ribonucleic acid
SA	Sinoatrial
SLE	Systemic lupus erythematosus
spp.	Species
SSRI	Selective serotonin reuptake inhibitor
SVT	Supraventricular tachycardia
TCA	Tricyclic antidepressant
TENS	Transcutaneous electrical nerve stimulation
TIBC	Total iron-binding capacity
TIVA	Total intravenous anaesthesia
tPA	tissue plasminogen activator
TSH	Thyroid-stimulating hormone
U&Es	Urea and electrolytes
UTI	Urinary tract infection
UVB	Ultraviolet B
VF	Ventricular fibrillation
VLDL	Very low–density lipoprotein
VRE	Vancomicin-resistant enterococci
VT	Ventricular tachycardia

CARDIOVASCULAR SYSTEM

Management guidelines (pp. 1–7)
Anaphylactic shock
Dysrhythmias
   Atrial fibrillation
      Paroxysmal
      Persistent
      Permanent
   Atrial flutter
   Supraventricular tachycardia
   Ventricular fibrillation
   Ventricular tachycardia
Heart failure
   Acute
   Chronic
Hyperlipidaemia
Hypertension
Ischaemic heart disease,
   Stable angina
   Unstable angina
   Myocardial infarction – ST elevation
   Post MI
Thromboembolism
   Deep vein thrombosis
   Pulmonary embolism

Drug classes (pp. 7–10)
ACE inhibitors
Beta blockers
Calcium channel blockers
Diuretics

Individual drugs (pp. 11–39)
Adenosine; Amiodarone; Amlodipine; Aspirin; Atenolol;
Atropine; Bendrofluazide; Bezafibrate; Clopidogrel; Digoxin;
Diltiazem; Dobutamine; Dopamine; Doxazosin; Epinephrine;
Furosemide; Heparin; Losartan; Methyldopa; Nicorandil;
Nitrates (GTN, ISDN, ISMN); Ramipril; Sildenafil;
Simvastatin; Tenecteplase; Verapamil; Warfarin

ANAPHYLACTIC SHOCK
• Give 0.5 mg (0.5 ml of 1 : 1000) epinephrine IM (given IV if there is no central pulse or if severely unwell)
• Give high-flow oxygen through face mask
• Gain IV access
• Give 10 mg of an antihistamine IV (e.g. chlorpheniramine)
• Give 100–200 mg hydrocortisone IV

- Consider salbutamol nebuliser and IV aminophylline if bronchospasm present
- Administer IV fluids if required to maintain BP
- Repeat epinephrine IM every 5 min if no improvement, as guided by BP, pulse and respiratory function
- If still no improvement, consider intubation and mechanical ventilation
- **Follow-up**:
  - Suggest a medic alert bracelet naming culprit allergen
  - Identify allergen with skin prick testing at a later stage
  - Self-injected epinephrine may be necessary for the future

DYSRHYTHMIAS
Atrial fibrillation (AF)
- Look for and treat any underlying cause
- **Paroxysmal AF**
  - Self-terminating, usually lasts less than 48 h
  - If recurrent, consider warfarin and antiarrhythmic drugs (e.g. sotalol, amiodarone)
- **Persistent AF**
  - Lasts more than 48 h and can be converted to sinus rhythm either chemically (amiodarone, sotalol or flecainide) or with synchronised D.C. shock
  - In cases of synchronised D.C. shock, administer warfarin for 1 month, then give D.C. shock under general anaesthetic to revert to sinus rhythm (only if no structural heart lesions are present) and continue warfarin for 1 month thereafter. If haemodynamically unstable, D.C. cardiovert without warfarin.
- **Permanent AF**
  - Digoxin for rate control and warfarin for anticoagulation (give aspirin if warfarin is contraindicated or inappropriate)
  - If digoxin fails, add or use a calcium channel blocker, beta blocker or amiodarone
  - Consider pacemaker if all else fails

Atrial flutter
- Look for and treat any underlying cause
- Treat as for acute AF
- In chronic atrial flutter maintain on warfarin and antiarrhythmic medication (e.g. sotalol, amiodarone)

Supraventricular tachycardia (SVT)
- Perform vagal manoeuvres (e.g. carotid sinus massage, immersion of the face in cold water)
- If this fails, give IV adenosine or IV verapamil
- If the patient is haemodynamically compromised, give synchronised D.C. shock under sedation or under short-acting GA (e.g. propofol)

- Other antiarrhythmics that can be tried are beta blockers, verapamil and amiodarone
- In chronic paroxysmal SVT consider regular antiarrhythmics (e.g. amiodarone, disopyramide) or electrical ablation of abnormal foci

Ventricular fibrillation (VF, pulseless VT)
- Protocols for the management of VF and pulseless VT are subject to constant updates. Consult current European Resuscitation Council or other appropriate guidelines.

Ventricular tachycardia with a pulse (VT)
- Look for and treat underlying causes and correct electrolyte imbalances
- Give IV lidocaine
- If this fails, give IV amiodarone or other antiarrhythmics or perform overdrive pacing
- Proceed to synchronised D.C. shock if patient is symptomatic, in cases of circulatory collapse or if there is no response to antiarrhythmic drugs
- Once recovered, consider implantable defibrillator or electrical ablation of abnormal foci

HEART FAILURE – ACUTE
- Sit the patient up
- Give 100% oxygen through face mask (24% in COPD)
- Give IV furosemide and GTN spray or tablet
- Give IV diamorphine with IV antiemetic (e.g. metoclopramide)
- If no improvement, consider IV GTN infusion (only if systolic BP > 100 mmHg)
- In cardiogenic shock (signified by falling BP) consider positive inotropes (dopamine, dobutamine) and intra-aortic balloon pump

HEART FAILURE – CHRONIC
- Treat any underlying cause (e.g. hypertension, valvular heart disease, IHD)
- Reduce salt intake and alter modifiable risk factors (e.g. smoking, obesity)
- If still symptomatic, give a loop diuretic (e.g. furosemide, bumetanide); a thiazide diuretic can be added (e.g. bendrofluazide or metalozone)
- If still symptomatic, add an ACE inhibitor (e.g. ramipril)
- If still no improvement, consider digoxin
- Vasodilators (e.g. hydralazine), oral nitrates (e.g. ISMN) and beta blockers (metoprolol, bisoprolol, carvedilol) can also be used

- Spironolactone (a potassium-sparing diuretic) has been shown to be of benefit in chronic heart failure
- Start warfarin to prevent thromboembolic events if AF is present or if there is significant cardiomegaly
- Consider cardiac transplant or biventricular pacing as a last resort (if patient meets criteria)
- Offer influenza vaccine

HYPERLIPIDAEMIA

- Advise weight reduction and decrease alcohol consumption if applicable
- Advise low-fat diet, substitute chicken and turkey for red meat and encourage fish, vegetables and fibre
- Treat any underlying causes of hyperlipidaemia: hypothyroidism, diabetes mellitus, chronic alcohol intake, drugs (e.g. thiazide diuretics, beta blockers)
- **Hypercholesterolaemia**: treat with an HMG CoA reductase inhibitor (e.g. simvastatin) if cholesterol levels > 5.5 mmol/L; treat regardless of lipid levels if IHD present
- Bile acid resins (e.g. cholestyramine), nicotinic acid, ezetimibe and fibrates can also be used to decrease cholesterol levels
- In **hypertriglyceridaemia**, fibrates (e.g. bezafibrate) are 1st line therapy but nicotinic acid can also be used
- In **mixed hyperlipidaemia** (high cholesterol and high triglycerides), statins or a combination of fibrates and statins can be used

HYPERTENSION

- Alter modifiable risk factors (e.g. smoking, obesity, alcohol, salt intake)
- Rule out secondary causes of hypertension (e.g. renal artery stenosis, Cushing's disease, coarctation of the aorta)
- Indications for treatment vary but generally treat if:
  - Systolic BP sustained > 160 mmHg or
  - Diastolic BP sustained > 100 mmHg
- Treat if diastolic BP 90–99 mmHg or systolic BP 140–159 mmHg in the presence of end-organ damage or if other risk factors (e.g. IHD, diabetes) present
- If BP 135–139/85–89 mmHg, reassess annually
- If BP < 135/85 mmHg, reassess 5-yearly

The following classes of antihypertensives are used in various combinations (tailored to the individual):

1 Thiazide diuretics (e.g. bendrofluazide)
2 Beta blockers (e.g. atenolol)
3 ACE inhibitors (e.g. captopril)
4 Calcium channel blockers (e.g. nifedipine)
5 Angiotensin II receptor antagonists (e.g. losartan)
6 Alpha blockers (e.g. doxazosin)
7 Centrally acting agents (e.g. methyldopa, moxonidine)

ISCHAEMIC HEART DISEASE
Stable angina
- Alter modifiable risk factors (smoking, hypertension, hyperlipidaemia, diabetes mellitus, obesity, diet, lack of exercise)
- 1st line therapy: sublingual GTN spray/tablet or skin patch for acute attacks
- Regular aspirin (if allergic or unable to tolerate aspirin, give clopidogrel)
- Maintenance therapy: beta blocker (e.g. atenolol)
- If still symptomatic, add a calcium channel blocker or a long-acting oral nitrate (isosorbide mononitrate or isosorbide dinitrate)
- If still symptomatic, give maintenance triple therapy (beta blocker, calcium channel blocker and a long-acting nitrate) + GTN for acute attacks
- *Note*: Do not give beta blockers with verapamil due to serious interactions
- Nicorandil, a potassium channel activator with vasodilator properties, is being increasingly used in the management of angina
- Last resort is coronary angioplasty or coronary bypass surgery

Unstable angina/non–ST elevation MI/non–Q wave MI
- Grouped together as acute coronary syndromes, since management is identical until blood results (cardiac enzymes) are known. These conditions are initially controlled medically and then investigated with a view to surgery or angioplasty.
- Give 100% oxygen through face mask (24% in COPD)
- Start regular oral aspirin (antiplatelet effect)
- Give oral clopidogrel (antiplatelet activity)
- Give subcutaneous low–molecular weight heparin or IV heparin (to prevent infarction in acute attack)
- Give IV nitrates (e.g. GTN), an oral beta blocker and an oral calcium channel blocker (e.g. amlodipine)
- If still symptomatic, start glycoprotein IIb/IIIa receptor antagonist (e.g. tirofiban – antiplatelet activity); usually started if intervention is anticipated, these drugs reduce events during and after PCI
- If still symptomatic, consider emergency coronary angioplasty or coronary bypass surgery

Myocardial infarction (ST elevation)
- Sit the patient up (to ease breathing and reduce venous return to the heart)
- Give 100% oxygen through face mask (24% in COPD)
- Attach cardiac monitor and perform 12-lead ECG
- Take blood for FBC, U&Es, cardiac enzymes, lipids and random glucose

- If patient is diabetic, commence on insulin sliding scale for 24 h, then subcutaneous insulin for 3 months post MI (if not already on insulin)
- For pain relief give IV diamorphine with IV antiemetic (e.g. metoclopramide)
- Limit infarct size:
  - Give aspirin (chewed or dissolved in water); if allergic to aspirin give clopidogrel
  - Give thrombolytic therapy if not contraindicated, preferably within 12 h following MI (streptokinase or tenecteplase)
- Give IV beta blocker if not contraindicated and if haemodynamically stable (aim to maintain heart rate of 55–65 beats per minute)
- Admit to coronary care unit
- Maintain serum potassium of 4–5 mmol/L to prevent cardiac dysrhythmias

Post myocardial infarction
- Heparin infusion or low–molecular weight heparin (enoxaparin or dalteparin) may be given to maintain vessel patency (usually for 5 days)
- If pain persists, IV nitrates (e.g. GTN) and diamorphine can be given
- If ST elevation persists, consider repeat thrombolysis or emergency angiogram with PCI or bypass surgery
- Look for and treat any complications:
  - Tachydysrhythmias – antiarrhythmic drugs, D.C. shock or overdrive pacing
  - Bradydysrhythmias – IV atropine, pacing
  - LVF with pulmonary oedema – IV furosemide followed by long-term ACE inhibitor
  - Cardiogenic shock – IV dopamine and IV dobutamine
  - Ventricular septal rupture/rupture of papillary muscle – urgent surgery
- Prevention of reinfarction:
  - Alter modifiable risk factors (smoking, obesity, hyperlipidaemia, hypertension, diabetes mellitus)
  - Daily aspirin for life, and a beta blocker (e.g. atenolol) for a minimum of 2–3 years
  - Long-term ACE inhibitor (e.g. ramipril) regardless of LV function
  - Add a statin (e.g. simvastatin)
- Advise no driving for 1 month and no work for 2 months
- Usually stay in CCU for 5 days
- ECG stress test on day 5:
  - If satisfactory, follow up in clinic 4–6 weeks later
  - If positive, or if ischaemic chest pain post MI, consider coronary angiogram and appropriate intervention with surgery or PCI as in- or outpatient

THROMBOEMBOLISM

Deep vein thrombosis
• Give IV or low–molecular weight subcutaneous heparin with oral warfarin
• Discontinue heparin when INR reaches therapeutic range
• Consider thrombolytic therapy (e.g. streptokinase) in cases of large thrombi
• Continue warfarin for a minimum of 3–6 months
• Look for and treat underlying cause
• Consider thrombophilia screen if no risk factors for DVT are present

Pulmonary embolism
• Perform investigations to help confirm diagnosis (d-dimer, ABGs, ECG, CXR, V/Q scan, CT pulmonary angiogram)
• Attach cardiac monitor
• Give 100% oxygen through face mask (24% in COPD)
• Give an NSAID for pleuritic pain
• For continuing pain, consider IV diamorphine + IV antiemetic (e.g. metoclopramide)
• Give an IV heparin loading dose followed by heparin infusion or low–molecular weight heparin
• Start oral warfarin at the same time as heparin and continue warfarin for 6 months (discontinue heparin when INR reaches therapeutic range)
• Consider thrombolytic therapy (e.g. streptokinase) if patient is haemodynamically unstable
• Look for and treat any underlying cause

Drug classes

ACE INHIBITORS
• Many types of ACE inhibitors exist, all of which have similar properties. They include captopril, lisinopril, enalapril, cilazapril, perindopril, quinapril and ramipril.

Indications
• Hypertension
• Heart failure
• Post MI
• Diabetic nephropathy

Note
• ACE inhibitors are generally well tolerated and have been shown to reduce mortality and morbidity in patients with heart failure (they are thought to prevent enlargement of the left

ventricle). Dry cough is a typical adverse effect and occurs in about 20% of patients taking ACE inhibitors.
• Angiotensin II receptor antagonists, such as losartan, have similar effects but their usefulness in heart failure has not yet been established.

BETA BLOCKERS
• There are two types of beta receptors: beta 1 and beta 2
• Beta 1 receptors are found in the heart
• Most other beta receptors are beta 2 receptors and are found in the peripheral vasculature, kidneys, skeletal muscle and airways

Types of Beta blockers
1 Selective (blocking beta 1 receptors): atenolol, bisoprolol and metoprolol
2 Non-selective (blocking both beta 1 and beta 2 receptors): nadolol, propranolol and timolol
• *Note*: Selective beta 1 blockers may also block beta 2 receptors to some extent, especially in high doses
• Beta blockers can also be either water-soluble, which are excreted renally unchanged (atenolol, celiprolol, nadolol, sotalol), or lipid-soluble, which are metabolised by the liver prior to excretion (metoprolol, propranolol)
• Some act as partial agonists (i.e. have ISA properties), such as celiprolol, oxprenolol and pindolol. They can simultaneously block and stimulate beta receptors. This results in less bradycardia and less peripheral vasoconstriction than with other beta blockers.
• Labetolol and carvedilol block both alpha and beta receptors

Indications
• Hypertension
• IHD
• Cardiac dysrhythmias
• Secondary prophylaxis in MI
• Heart failure

Non-selective beta blockers can further be used in:
• Thyrotoxicosis (for symptom control)
• Prophylaxis of migraine
• Glaucoma
• Anxiety (for prevention of palpitations, tremor and tachycardia)
• Essential tremor
• Secondary prophylaxis of oesophageal varices

Effects
Beta blockers can cause the following effects:
• Beta 1 receptor blockade – decreased force of myocardial contraction and decreased heart rate

- Beta 2 receptor blockade in the kidneys – decreased renin release and hence lowered BP
- Beta 2 receptor blockade in skeletal muscle – tiredness
- Beta 2 receptor blockade in the airways – bronchospasm
- Beta 2 receptor blockade in blood vessels– peripheral vasoconstriction (i.e. cold extremities)
- Lipid-soluble beta blockers cross the blood–brain barrier and can cause sleep disturbance and nightmares (this also applies to water-soluble beta blockers, but to a lesser extent)

CALCIUM CHANNEL BLOCKERS
Types of calcium channel blockers
1 Dihydropyridines: amlodipine, felodipine, nicardipine, nifedipine, nimodipine, nisoldipine, isradipine
2 Phenylalkalamines: verapamil
3 Benzothiazepines: diltiazem

Indications
- Hypertension
- Angina
- Supraventricular dysrhythmias (verapamil or diltiazem)

Mechanism of action
- All calcium channel blockers act on L-type calcium channels at different sites:
  - Myocardium
  - The conducting system of the heart
  - Vascular smooth muscle

Dihydropyridines
- Dihydropyridines act mainly on peripheral and coronary vasculature and are therefore used to treat angina (usually combined with a beta blocker)
- Dihydropyridines can be used alone in the treatment of hypertension or can be safely combined with a beta blocker
- Dihydropyridines have very few cardiac effects

Verapamil and diltiazem
- Verapamil and diltiazem act both on the heart and on peripheral blood vessels. They decrease heart rate, force of contraction and have antiarrhythmic properties. They also cause peripheral vasodilatation and dilatation of coronary arteries.
- Verapamil and diltiazem must be used with extreme caution if given with beta blockers, due to hazardous interactions such as asystole and AV node block

DIURETICS

Types of diuretics

1 Thiazides: bendrofluazide, benzthiazide, chlorthalidone, clopamide, cyclopenthiazide, hydrochlorothiazide, hydroflumethiazide, indapamide, metalozone, xipamide
2 Loop diuretics: furosemide, bumetanide, torasemide
3 Potassium-sparing: spironolactone, amiloride, triamterene
4 Carbonic anhydrase inhibitors: acetazolamide, dorzolamide
5 Osmotic: mannitol

Indications

- Hypertension (thiazides)
- Chronic heart failure (loop diuretics, thiazides or in combination)
- Oedema (loop diuretics, thiazides or in combination)
- Glaucoma (acetazolamide, dorzolamide or mannitol)
- Raised intracranial pressure (mannitol)

Note

- Loop diuretics are the most effective diuretics, followed by thiazides.
- Potassium-sparing diuretics are weak and not normally used on their own. They are usually given with loop diuretics or thiazides to prevent hypokalaemia.
- Potassium-sparing diuretics should not normally be used with ACE inhibitors as dangerous hyperkalaemia may result.
- Loop and thiazide diuretics act synergistically and are effective in the treatment of resistant oedema.

Adenosine

Class: Antiarrhythmic agent

Indications
- Paroxysmal supraventricular dysrhythmias
- To differentiate between SVT with aberrant conduction and VT

Mechanism of action
- Adenosine acts on the SA and AV nodes by binding to adenosine receptors in the conducting tissue of the heart and by activating potassium channels. This slows conduction in the heart and causes a decrease in the heart rate.

Adverse effects
- *Common*: chest pain, bronchospasm, flushing, light-headedness, nausea (all transient, usually lasting a few seconds)
- *Rare*: severe bradycardia, transient asystole, hypotension

Contraindications
- Asthma
- 2nd or 3rd degree heart block (unless pacemaker in situ)
- Sick sinus syndrome

Interactions
- *Dipyridamole*: this enhances adenosine effects
- *Theophylline*: this inhibits the action of adenosine by blocking adenosine receptors

Route of administration
- IV

Note
- Prior to administration of adenosine the patient should be warned about the transient adverse effects such as chest pain, as they may cause great distress.
- Adenosine has a very short duration of action (about 8 seconds), therefore adverse effects are mostly short-lived.

Amiodarone

Class: Antiarrhythmic agent

Indications
- Supraventricular dysrhythmias
- Ventricular dysrhythmias (including VF and pulseless VT in cardiac arrest)

Mechanism of action
- Amiodarone prolongs the refractory period in all parts of the conducting system of the heart. This decreases the speed of impulses moving through the heart.
- Amiodarone also has some beta-blocking and some weak calcium channel–blocking properties.

Adverse effects
- *Common*: reversible corneal deposits (in long-term use), photosensitive rash
- *Rare*: hypo- or hyperthyroidism, pulmonary fibrosis, hepatitis, neurological symptoms (e.g. tremor, ataxia), peripheral neuropathy, grey skin colour, metallic taste in the mouth, myopathy

Contraindications
- Cardiac conduction defects (e.g. sick sinus syndrome)
- Thyroid disease
- Pregnancy
- Breastfeeding
- Iodine allergy (as amiodarone contains iodine)

Interactions
- *Beta blockers*: concomitant use of amiodarone and beta blockers increases the risk of AV block, bradycardia and myocardial depression
- *Digoxin*: amiodarone increases the plasma concentration of digoxin
- *Diltiazem, verapamil*: concomitant use of amiodarone with diltiazem or verapamil increases the risk of AV block, bradycardia and myocardial depression
- *Phenytoin*: amiodarone inhibits the metabolism of phenytoin
- *Warfarin*: amiodarone enhances the effect of warfarin by inhibiting its metabolism

Route of administration
- Oral, IV

Note
- Thyroid function and LFTs should be monitored every 6 months whilst on treatment with amiodarone.
- Pulmonary function tests should be performed prior to and during treatment with amiodarone in order to detect any developing pulmonary fibrosis.
- Patients should be advised to use sunblock to prevent photosensitivity rash.
- Amiodarone has a half-life of about 36 days and therefore interactions can occur long after the drug has been stopped.

Amlodipine

Class: Calcium channel blocker

Indications
- Hypertension
- Prophylaxis and treatment of angina

Mechanism of action
- Amlodipine inhibits the influx of calcium into vascular smooth muscle (and, to a lesser extent, into myocardium) by binding to the L-type calcium channels, especially in arterioles. This results in relaxation of vascular smooth muscle with a subsequent decrease in peripheral resistance and BP.
- Amlodipine dilates coronary arteries, which contributes to its antianginal effect.

Adverse effects
- *Common*: headache, flushing, ankle swelling, dizziness
- *Rare*: urinary frequency, GI disturbances, mood changes, palpitations, impotence

Contraindications
- Pregnancy and breastfeeding
- Cardiogenic shock
- Advanced aortic stenosis
- Unstable angina

Interactions
- *Antihypertensives*: amlodipine increases the hypotensive effect

Route of administration
- Oral

Note
- Amlodipine can be safely used in asthmatics, for whom beta blockers are contraindicated.
- For best effect in severe angina, amlodipine should be combined with a beta blocker.

Related drugs
- Other dihydropyridine calcium channel blockers: felodipine, isradipine, lacidipine, lercanidipine, nicardipine, nifedipine, nimodipine, nisoldipine

Aspirin

Class: Non-steroidal anti-inflammatory drug (NSAID)

Indications
- Prophylaxis of MI, ischaemic stroke, transient ischaemic attacks
- Mild to moderate pain and inflammation
- Pyrexia

Mechanism of action
- Aspirin irreversibly inhibits the enzymes COX-1 and COX-2. This leads to the inhibition of prostaglandin synthesis and hence to:
  1. a decrease in vascular permeability and vasodilatation (anti-inflammatory effect);
  2. a decrease in sensitisation of pain afferents (analgesic effect); and
  3. a decrease in the effect of prostaglandins on the hypothalamus (antipyretic effect).
- Platelets contain a high concentration of cyclo-oxygenase 1 (COX-1), which is necessary for thromboxane A_2 production. Aspirin inhibits this process and hence inhibits thrombus formation (antiplatelet effect).

Adverse effects
- *Common*: GI irritation (gastritis, gastric ulcer, bleeding), bleeding tendency
- *Rare*: bronchospasm, rash, thrombocytopenia, renal failure

Contraindications
- Children under 16 (as aspirin may cause Reye's syndrome) except when specifically indicated (e.g. juvenile arthritis)
- Previous or active peptic ulcer
- Gout (aspirin inhibits uric acid excretion)
- Bleeding disorders (e.g. haemophilia)
- Breastfeeding
- History of hypersensitivity

Interactions
- *SSRIs*: concomitant use of aspirin and SSRIs increases the risk of bleeding
- *Warfarin*: concomitant use of aspirin and warfarin increases the risk of bleeding

Route of administration
- Oral, rectal

Note
- The risk of gastric irritation can be reduced by taking aspirin after food or by using the enteric-coated form.
- In high doses aspirin can lead to salicylate intoxication (dizziness, tinnitus, deafness).
- Aspirin is associated with Reye's syndrome in children under 16 years of age (a condition characterised by encephalitis and liver failure). Paracetamol is thus the preferred option in this age group.

Atenolol

Class: Beta blocker

Indications
- Hypertension
- Angina
- Supraventricular dysrhythmias
- Secondary prophylaxis of MI

Mechanism of action
- Atenolol reduces heart rate and force of myocardial contraction by acting on beta 1 receptors in the heart. This results in decreased workload of the heart; hence its use in angina.
- Renin production by the kidney is also reduced by atenolol, which contributes to its antihypertensive effect.
- Atenolol decreases the effects of sympathetic activity on the heart with a resulting decrease in conduction and in action potential initiation; hence its use as an antiarrythmic.

Adverse effects
- *Common*: lethargy (usually ceases after long-term use), bradycardia and AV block, hypotension, cold peripheries
- *Rare*: bronchospasm, worsened or precipitated heart failure, nightmares, impotence

Contraindications
- Asthma
- Uncontrolled heart failure (including cardiogenic shock)
- Cardiac conduction defects (e.g. 2nd and 3rd degree heart block)
- Bradycardia
- COPD
- Metabolic acidosis
- Hypotension

Interactions
- *Diltiazem*: concomitant use of diltiazem and atenolol increases the risk of bradycardia and AV block
- *Verapamil*: the risk of heart failure, severe hypotension and asystole is increased if atenolol is given with verapamil

Route of administration
- Oral, IV

Note
- Atenolol is selective for beta 1 receptors, but at high doses it can also block beta 2 receptors, thus causing bronchospasm.
- Abrupt withdrawal of atenolol may worsen angina.
- Beta blockers may mask the symptoms of hypoglycaemia caused by oral hypoglycaemics or insulin.

Related drugs
- Bisoprolol, carvedilol, celiprolol, esmolol, labetolol, metoprolol, nadolol, oxprenolol, pindolol, propranolol, sotalol, timolol

Atropine

Class: Muscarinic antagonist

Indications
- Cardiac arrest
- Bradycardia
- Organophosphorus poisoning
- For paralysis of the ciliary muscle (allowing measurement of the refractive error in children)
- Anterior uveitis
- Irritable bowel syndrome

Mechanism of action
- Atropine decreases the activity of the parasympathetic nervous system by blocking the action of acetylcholine on muscarinic receptors. This leads to pupillary dilatation, bronchodilatation, increase in heart rate and decreased secretions from sweat, salivary and bronchial glands.
- Atropine also reduces gut motility and bronchial secretions.

Adverse effects
- *Common*: antimuscarinic effects (e.g. dry mouth, blurred vision, constipation, dilated pupils)
- *Rare*: confusion (especially in the elderly), palpitations, irritation of the eye (when given as eye drops), acute urinary retention

Contraindications
- Prostatic hypertrophy
- Closed-angle glaucoma
- Paralytic ileus
- Myasthenia gravis
- Pyloric stenosis

Interactions
- *TCAs, MAOIs and antihistamines*: increased risk of antimuscarinic side-effects

Route of administration
- Oral (rarely used for irritable bowel syndrome), IV (bradycardia, cardiac arrest), IM (organophosphorus poisoning), eye drops

Note
- Atropine can be used to reverse the adverse effects of neostigmine (e.g. excessive bradycardia). In this case it is given IV.
- When used in anterior uveitis, aim of treatment is to prevent complications.
- Occasionally atropine is given with anaesthetics such as propofol, halothane and suxamethonium to prevent bradycardia and hypotension during general anaesthesia.
- Atropine is also used to decrease salivary and bronchial secretions that are increased during intubation prior to surgery.

Related drugs
- Hyoscine hydrobromide

Bendrofluazide

Class: Thiazide diuretic

Indications
- Hypertension
- Heart failure
- Oedema secondary to liver disease, nephrotic syndrome, low protein diet or heart failure
- Prophylaxis of calcium-containing renal stones

Mechanism of action
- Bendrofluazide acts on the proximal part of the distal tubule in the nephron where it inhibits Na^+ and Cl^- reabsorption. This leads to increased excretion of Na^+, Cl^- and water, which stimulates potassium excretion further down in the distal tubule. All these events lead to hypokalaemia, hyponatraemia and a decrease in intravascular volume.
- Reduced intravascular volume causes an initial decrease in cardiac output (hence initial antihypertensive effect), but a reduction in peripheral resistance is responsible for lowering BP in the long term.

Adverse effects
- *Common*: hypokalaemia, dehydration, postural hypotension
- *Rare*: impotence, hyperuricaemia, hyperglycaemia, hyperlipidaemia, hypercalcaemia, thrombocytopenia, hyponatraemia, photosensitivity, pancreatitis

Contraindications
- Hypokalaemia, hyponatraemia, hypercalcaemia
- Severe hepatic and renal impairment
- Gout
- Addison's disease

Interactions
- *Digoxin*: hypokalaemia caused by bendrofluazide potentiates the effects of digoxin
- *Lithium*: bendrofluazide increases the plasma concentration of lithium

Route of administration
- Oral

Note
- Low doses of bendrofluazide cause minimal biochemical disturbance and are fully effective at lowering BP. Higher doses do not decrease BP any further, but make biochemical adverse effects more likely.
- Prolonged use at high doses may lead to hypokalaemia, which may cause cardiac dysrhythmias (hence potassium levels must be monitored). If high doses are prescribed, it is recommended to combine bendrofluazide with either potassium supplements, a potassium-sparing diuretic (e.g. amiloride) or an ACE inhibitor.

Related drugs
- Chlorthalidone, cyclopenthiazide, hydrochlorothiazide, indapamide, metalozone, xipamide

Bezafibrate

Class: Fibrate

Indications
- Hyperlipidaemia

Mechanism of action
- Bezafibrate reduces triglyceride levels by stimulating the enzyme lipoprotein lipase, which converts triglycerides into fatty acids and glycerol.
- Bezafibrate also reduces cholesterol levels (to a lesser extent than triglycerides) by reducing cholesterol production in the liver. It decreases circulating LDL levels and also increases the levels of beneficial HDL.

Adverse effects
- *Common*: nausea, abdominal discomfort, headache
- *Rare*: myositis syndrome (muscle pain, stiffness, weakness), impotence, rash, pruritus, gallstones

Contraindications
- Hepatic impairment
- Pregnancy and breastfeeding
- Nephrotic syndrome
- Gallbladder disease
- Primary biliary cirrhosis

Interactions
- *HMG CoA reductase inhibitors*: concomitant use of bezafibrate and HMG CoA reductase inhibitors increases the risk of myositis syndrome
- *Warfarin*: bezafibrate potentiates the anticoagulant effect of warfarin by displacing it from plasma protein binding sites

Route of administration
- Oral

Note
- Drug treatment of hyperlipidaemia is recommended when patients fail to respond to dietary measures.
- It has been shown that fibrates are less effective than statins in the prevention of cardiovascular events (e.g. MI).

Related drugs
- Ciprofibrate, fenofibrate, gemfibrozil

Clopidogrel

Class: Antiplatelet drug

Indications
• Prevention of vascular events after ischaemic stroke, after MI and in peripheral vascular disease
• Acute coronary syndromes

Mechanism of action
• Clopidogrel irreversibly modifies ADP receptors on platelets and thus prevents ADP from binding to them. This prevents activation of glycoprotein GpIIB/IIIa complex and therefore prevents platelet aggregation.
• Platelets exposed to clopidogrel are affected for the rest of their lifespan, which is 8–10 days.

Adverse effects
• *Rare*: bleeding (GI tract, intracranial), abdominal pain, diarrhoea, peptic ulcers, neutropenia, thrombotic thrombocytopenic purpura, hepatic impairment

Contraindications
• Active bleeding
• Breastfeeding

Interactions
• *Anticoagulants/other antiplatelet drugs*: these increase the risk of bleeding
• *NSAIDs*: these increase the risk of bleeding

Route of administration
• Oral

Note
• Clopidogrel is used when aspirin is contraindicated or not tolerated.
• Clopidogrel can be added to aspirin in the treatment of acute coronary syndromes for a more effective antiplatelet effect.

Related drugs
• Other antiplatelet drugs: abciximab, aspirin, dipyridamole, eptifibatide, tirofiban

Digoxin

Class: Cardiac glycoside

Indications
- Supraventricular dysrhythmias
- Heart failure

Mechanism of action
- The primary action of digoxin on the heart is to inhibit the Na^+/K^+ ATP pump. This increases intracellular Na^+ concentration, which in turn inhibits the Na^+/Ca^{2+} exchanger and hence the amount of calcium pumped out of the cell. These events lead to increased intracellular calcium in myocardial cells, which increases the force of myocardial contraction.
- Digoxin slows the heart rate by increasing vagal activity. It also slows conduction through the AV node (hence its use in dysrhythmias).

Adverse effects
- *Common*: nausea, vomiting, anorexia, diarrhoea, digoxin toxicity in overdose (e.g. cardiac dysrhythmias)
- *Rare*: gynaecomastia in chronic use, confusion, hallucinations, yellow vision

Contraindications
- 2nd degree heart block
- Hypertrophic obstructive cardiomyopathy
- Wolff–Parkinson–White syndrome

Interactions
- *Amiodarone, propafenone, quinidine*: these antiarrhythmic drugs increase the risk of digoxin toxicity
- *Diltiazem, nicardipine, verapamil*: these increase the risk of digoxin toxicity

Route of administration
- Oral, IV (for emergency loading dose)

Note
- In heart failure, digoxin does not reduce mortality but improves symptoms and reduces the frequency of hospital admissions at the expense of possible digoxin toxicity.
- Digoxin has a narrow therapeutic window and therefore requires therapeutic drug monitoring.
- The risk of digoxin toxicity is greater in hypokalaemia. Patients receiving digoxin and potassium-losing diuretics may therefore require potassium supplements or a potassium-sparing diuretic.
- Hypomagnesaemia, hypercalcaemia and hypothyroidism also increase the risk of digoxin toxicity.

Related drugs
- Digitoxin

Diltiazem

Class: Calcium channel blocker

Indications
- Prophylaxis and treatment of angina
- Hypertension

Mechanism of action
- Diltiazem inhibits the influx of calcium into vascular smooth muscle and myocardium by binding to the L-type calcium channels. This results in:
  1 relaxation of vascular smooth muscle with subsequent decrease in peripheral resistance and BP;
  2 decreased myocardial contractility; and
  3 slowed conduction at the AV node and prolonged refractory period (hence its use as an antiarrhythmic).
- Reduction in afterload, myocardial contractility and heart rate lead to reduced oxygen consumption, thereby relieving angina.

Adverse effects
- *Common*: headache, nausea, dizziness, hypotension, bradycardia, ankle swelling
- *Rare*: lethargy, rash, AV block

Contraindications
- Severe bradycardia
- 2nd and 3rd degree heart block
- Sick sinus syndrome
- Heart failure
- Pregnancy and breastfeeding

Interactions
- *Antiarrhythmics*: diltiazem may potentiate the myocardial depression caused by other antiarrhythmic drugs
- *Beta blockers*: these increase the risk of AV block and bradycardia if given with diltiazem
- *Digoxin*: diltiazem increases the plasma concentration of digoxin
- *Theophylline*: diltiazem enhances the effects of theophylline

Route of administration
- Oral

Note
- Diltiazem can be used in patients with coronary artery spasm (Prinzmetal's angina).
- Diltiazem has the fewest adverse effects of all calcium channel blockers.
- It has a short half-life due to extensive first-pass metabolism.

Related drugs
- Verapamil

Dobutamine

Class: Inotropic sympathomimetic

Indications
- Inotropic support in the following:
  - Cardiogenic shock
  - Cardiac surgery
  - Septic shock
- Pharmacological cardiac stress testing

Mechanism of action
- Dobutamine stimulates beta 1 receptors in the heart. This results in increased cardiac contractility.
- Unlike dopamine, dobutamine does not cause release of norepinephrine.

Adverse effects
- *Common*: tachycardia (dobutamine has a lesser tendency to cause tachycardia than dopamine), temporary premature ventricular beats, temporary rise in BP
- *Rare*: cardiac dysrhythmias, shortness of breath

Contraindications
- None
- Caution:
  - Severe hypotension

Interactions
- *Beta blockers*: severe hypertension may occur

Route of administration
- IV

Note
- Dobutamine does not reduce renal perfusion and for this reason is preferred to beta agonists in the treatment of shock.
- Dobutamine is often combined with low dose dopamine in the treatment of cardiogenic shock.

Related drugs
- Dopamine, dopexamine

Dopamine

Class: Inotropic sympathomimetic

Indications
- Cardiogenic shock following MI
- Hypotension following cardiac surgery
- Initiation of diuresis in chronic heart failure

Mechanism of actiono
- The actions of dopamine are dose-dependent.
- In low doses ($< 5\,\mu g/kg/min$), dopamine acts on dopamine receptors resulting in renal, coronary and mesenteric vasodilatation. This improves perfusion in those areas.
- In moderate doses (5–$20\,\mu g/kg/min$), dopamine increases cardiac contractility and causes tachycardia by acting on cardiac beta 1 adrenoceptors.
- In high doses ($> 20\,\mu g/kg/min$), dopamine causes vasoconstriction by acting on alpha adrenoceptors.

Adverse effects
- *Common*:
  - Low doses: nausea, vomiting
  - Moderate to high doses: tachycardia, ventricular ectopic beats, peripheral vasoconstriction, hypotension or hypertension

Contraindications
- Untreated tachydysrhythmias
- Phaeochromocytoma

Interactions
- *MAOIs*: dopamine can cause a hypertensive crisis if given with MAOIs

Route of administration
- IV

Note
- Moderate and high doses of dopamine must be administered through a central venous line.
- BP, heart rate and urine output must be monitored during treatment.
- Dopamine should not be infused into alkaline solutions as this would render it inactive.
- Extravasation of dopamine can cause skin necrosis. If this occurs, phentolamine should be infiltrated into the ischaemic area. This neutralises dopamine.

Related drugs
- Dobutamine, dopexamine

Doxazosin

Class: Alpha 1 blocker

Indications
- Hypertension
- Benign prostatic hyperplasia

Mechanism of action
- Doxazosin inhibits beta 1–mediated vasoconstriction, thus causing reduction in peripheral resistance with a subsequent fall in blood pressure.
- Doxazosin also relaxes smooth muscle in the internal urethral sphincter resulting in increased urinary outflow in BPH.

Adverse effects
- *Common*: postural hypotension, dizziness, headache, GI upset, fatigue
- *Rare*: impotence, flu-like symptoms, rash

Contraindications
- Heart failure
- Caution:
  - Hepatic impairment
  - Pregnancy
  - Breastfeeding

Interactions
- *Antidepressants*: doxazosin enhances the hypotensive effect of antidepressants
- *Beta blockers*: doxazosin enhances the hypotensive effect of beta blockers
- *Calcium channel blockers*: doxazosin enhances the hypotensive effect of calcium channel blockers
- *Diuretics*: doxazosin enhances the hypotensive effect of diuretics

Route of administration
- Oral

Note
- Long-term therapy with doxazosin lowers plasma LDL, VLDL and triglyceride levels. It also increases HDL levels and is therefore considered beneficial in patients with CHD.

Related drugs
- Indoramin, prazosin, terazosin

Epinephrine (adrenaline)

Class: Sympathomimetic agent

Indications
- Anaphylaxis
- Cardiac arrest
- Prolongation of the effects of local anaesthetics
- Open-angle glaucoma
- Severe asthma and croup

Mechanism of action
- Epinephrine has various effects due to stimulation of the sympathetic nervous system. It is a potent alpha and beta receptor agonist. It is more beta 2 selective, but does not distinguish between alpha 1 and alpha 2 receptors.
- Beta 1 receptor stimulation increases the heart rate and force of myocardial contraction. Beta 2 receptor stimulation results in vasodilatation, bronchodilatation and uterine relaxation.
- Alpha receptor stimulation causes vasoconstriction, which prolongs the action of local anaesthetics by preventing their spread from the site of application.
- In anaphylactic shock, epinephrine raises BP and causes bronchodilatation.
- Epinephrine is thought to decrease the production of aqueous humor and increase its outflow from the anterior chamber of the eye; hence its use in glaucoma.
- In asthma and croup, epinephrine reduces bronchial muscle spasm and decreases airway swelling, respectively.

Adverse effects
- *Common*: anxiety, restlessness, tremor, tachycardia, hypertension
- *Rare*: cardiac dysrhythmias, cerebral haemorrhage, pulmonary oedema (all in overdose)

Contraindications
- Closed-angle glaucoma

Interactions
- *Beta blockers*: these can cause severe hypertension if given with epinephrine
- *Tricyclic antidepressants*: these increase the risk of cardiac dysrhythmias and hypertension if given with epinephrine

Route of administration
- IM (anaphylactic shock), IV (cardiac arrest), subcutaneous (with local anaesthetics), inhalation (asthma, croup), eye drops

Note
- Epinephrine is frequently administered with local anaesthetics (e.g. lidocaine) except in the fingers, toes and penis where prolonged vasoconstriction may result in gangrene.
- In CPR, epinephrine can be given through an endotracheal tube if IV access is unobtainable. In this case the dose should be doubled.

Furosemide (frusemide)

Class: Loop diuretic

Indications
- Acute and chronic heart failure
- Fluid overload
- Oedema
- Hypercalcaemia

Mechanism of action
- Furosemide inhibits reabsorption of Na^+, K^+ and water in the ascending limb of the loop of Henle in the kidneys by inhibiting the $Na^+/K^+/2Cl^-$ pump at this site. This leads to increased salt, water and potassium loss.
- Furosemide further decreases preload by causing venodilatation. This reduces ventricular filling pressures in the heart.
- It also reduces CSF production.

Adverse effects
- *Common*: postural hypotension, hypokalaemia, hyponatraemia, hyperuricaemia and gout
- *Rare*: bone marrow suppression, GI disturbance, reversible deafness (only in high doses or in patients with renal failure), hypocalcaemia, pancreatitis

Contraindications
- Renal failure with anuria

Interactions
- *Antibacterials*: furosemide increases the risk of ototoxity associated with aminoglycosides and vancomicin
- *Digoxin*: furosemide-induced hypokalaemia enhances the effects of digoxin, thus increasing the risk of digoxin-induced dysrhythmias
- *Lithium*: furosemide decreases lithium excretion, leading to an increased risk of lithium toxicity
- *NSAIDs*: concomitant use increases the risk of nephrotoxicity

Route of administration
- Oral, IM, IV

Note
- Furosemide causes potassium loss. A potassium-sparing diuretic (e.g. amiloride), potassium supplements or an ACE inhibitor should be prescribed with it.
- Loop diuretics are more effective than thiazide diuretics.

Related drugs
- Bumetanide, torasemide

Heparin

Class: Anticoagulant

Indications
- Prophylaxis and treatment of deep vein thrombosis
- Pulmonary embolism
- Unstable angina
- Myocardial infarction
- Acute occlusion of peripheral arteries
- Extracorporeal circuits (e.g. haemodialysis, cardiopulmonary bypass)

Mechanism of action
- Heparin potentiates the action of antithrombin III, which inactivates thrombin and other clotting factors (especially Xa) involved in the clotting pathway. This inhibits thrombus formation.
- Heparin has an antiplatelet effect by binding to and inhibiting von Willebrand factor.

Adverse effects
- *Common*: haemorrhage, thrombocytopenia
- *Rare*: osteoporosis or alopecia with long-term use, skin necrosis, rash, anaphylaxis

Contraindications
- Haemorrhage
- Haemophilia/thrombocytopenia
- Peptic ulceration
- Following major trauma
- Recent haemorrhagic stroke or recent surgery
- Severe hypertension
- Severe liver disease

Interactions
- *Aspirin and clopidogrel*: both increase the risk of haemorrhage if given with heparin
- *Glyceryl trinitrate*: a GTN infusion increases the excretion of heparin

Route of administration
- IV, subcutaneous

Note
- Two types of heparin are available: unfractionated heparin and low–molecular weight heparin. They are both of equal efficacy, but low–molecular weight heparin has a longer duration of action (e.g. dalteparin).
- Low–molecular weight heparin is preferred to unfractionated heparin because it can be given subcutaneously and avoids the need for APTT monitoring.
- Treatment with heparin must be monitored by measuring the APTT, preferably on a daily basis.
- The effects of heparin can be reversed by IV protamine sulphate injection.

Related drugs
- Other low–molecular weight heparins: certoparin, dalteparin, enoxaparin, reviparin, tinzaparin

Losartan

Class: Angiotensin II receptor blocker

Indications
- Hypertension
- Diabetic nephropathy in type 2 diabetes mellitus

Mechanism of action
- Losartan is a reversible competitive antagonist at angiotensin II receptors (confusingly known as AT1 receptors), which are found in vascular smooth muscle and in the adrenal glands. This action blocks the vasoconstrictor effects of angiotensin II, and it reduces aldosterone secretion from the adrenal cortex. These actions in turn result in an antihypertensive effect.
- Losartan does not inhibit ACE. See also *Mechanism of action* of Ramipril.

Adverse effects
- *Common*: headaches, dizziness, diarrhoea
- *Rare*: myalgia, vasculits, hepatitis, taste disturbance, hyperkalaemia, rash, pruritus

Contraindications
- Breastfeeding
- Pregnancy

Interactions
- *Ciclosporin*: risk of hyperkalaemia
- *ACE inhibitors*: risk of hyperkalaemia
- *Potassium-sparing diuretics*: risk of hyperkalaemia

Route of administration
- Oral

Note
- Losartan does not have an effect on bradykinin and other kinins and therefore does not cause a dry cough to the extent that ACE inhibitors do.
- Losartan is effective in reducing progression of renal disease in diabetic patients, independent of lowering the blood pressure.
- Currently only losartan and valsartan can be used to prevent renal failure in type 2 diabetes.

Related drugs
- Candesartan, eprosartan, irbesartan, olmesartan, telmisartan, valsartan

Methyldopa

Class: Centrally acting antihypertensive agent

Indications
- Hypertension

Mechanism of action
- Methyldopa is converted to its active component, alpha-methylnorepinephrine, within adrenergic nerve endings. This compound stimulates alpha 2 adrenoceptors of the vasomotor centre in the medulla, causing reduced sympathetic outflow. Subsequently, this leads to vasodilatation and a fall in blood pressure.

Adverse effects
- *Common*: drowsiness, headache, postural hypotension, depression, impotence
- *Rare*: haemolytic anaemia, diarrhoea, nasal congestion, hepatitis, gynaecomastia

Contraindications
- Depression
- Active hepatic disease
- Porphyria
- Phaeochromocytoma

Interactions
- *Anaesthetics*: these enhance the hypotensive effect of methyldopa
- *Antidepressants*: these enhance the hypotensive effect of methyldopa
- *Ciclosporin*: increased risk of myositis
- *Lithium*: concomitant use of methyldopa and lithium may cause neurotoxicity

Route of administration
- Oral, IV

Note
- Methyldopa is commonly prescribed for hypertension in pregnancy. It crosses the placenta and appears in breast milk but has no adverse effects on the fetus.
- Treatment with methyldopa may result in a positive Direct Coombs Test.

Related drugs
- Clonidine, moxonidine

Nicorandil

Class: Potassium channel activator

Indications
- Prevention and treatment of stable angina

Mechanism of action
- Nicorandil's action includes both nitrate-like effects and activation of ATP-sensitive potassium channels in vascular smooth muscle. This leads to vasodilatation in coronary, arterial and venous systems, which in turn reduces preload, afterload and myocardial oxygen consumption.
- Nicorandil has no significant effects on myocardial contractility.

Adverse effects
- *Common*: headache, nausea, vomiting, dizziness, facial flushing
- *Rare*: angina, palpitations, mouth ulcers, myalgia, angioedema, bronchitis, dyspnoea

Contraindications
- Cardiogenic shock
- Hypotension
- LVF

Interactions
- *MAOIs*: these enhance the hypotensive effect
- *Sildenafil*: this enhances the hypotensive effect

Route of administration
- Oral

Note
- Headaches usually diminish with continued use.
- Nicorandil has been shown to reduce the incidence of ventricular/supraventricular tachycardias and myocardial ischaemia in patients already on maximum conventional antianginal therapy. This effect is believed to be due to nicorandil mimicking the natural process of ischaemic preconditioning, whereby the heart's inbuilt mechanism makes it more and more resistant to ischaemic episodes.
- Nicorandil is currently the only potassium channel activator in use.

Nitrates (glyceryl trinitrate, isosorbide mononitrate, isosorbide dinitrate)

Class: Organic nitrates

Indications
- Angina
- Heart failure
- Malignant hypertension
- Anal fissure (applied as GTN ointment)

Mechanism of action
- Nitrates are metabolised into nitric oxide within vascular smooth muscle cells. This compound causes relaxation of vascular smooth muscle through activation of guanylyl cyclase. As a result, coronary arteries and systemic veins vasodilate, with ensuing decrease in preload and improved oxygen supply to the myocardium.
- Nitrates also reduce afterload to some extent. This is useful in the treatment of heart failure.

Adverse effects
- *Common*: headache, dizziness, postural hypotension, flushing, tachycardia

Contraindications
- Hypotension or hypovolaemia
- Aortic or mitral stenosis
- Constrictive pericarditis
- Cardiac tamponade
- HOCM
- Closed-angle glaucoma

Interactions
- *Sildenafil*: this enhances the hypotensive effect of nitrates

Route of administration
- Sublingual, skin patch or skin ointment (all for angina), IV (for unstable angina, acute heart failure, malignant hypertension), oral (for angina, heart failure)

Note
- Sublingual GTN or a GTN skin patch can be used prophylactically before exercise to prevent angina.
- Properties of isosorbide dinitrate and isosorbide mononitrate are similar to those of GTN but they can be taken orally and have a longer duration of action (several hours).
- Tolerance to long-acting nitrates (ISDN and ISMN) develops after as little as 24 h of continued administration. Their effects thus become progressively weaker. This can be minimised by allowing drug-free periods of 8 h.

Ramipril

Class: Angiotensin-converting enzyme inhibitor

Indications
- Hypertension
- Heart failure
- Post MI
- Diabetic nephropathy

Mechanism of action
- Ramipril inhibits ACE, leading to decreased synthesis of angiotensin II. This results in an antihypertensive effect largely due to:
  - Vasodilatation (angiotensin II is a vasoconstrictor);
  - Reduced levels of aldosterone and hence reduced sodium and water retention; and
  - Accumulation of bradykinin (a vasodilator).
- Ramipril prevents glomerular injury by angiotensin II in the kidneys.
- Ramipril is also thought to
  - prevent atherogenesis and thrombosis in blood vessels; and
  - prevent left ventricular hypertrophy and dysfunction.

Adverse effects
- *Common*: postural hypotension, dry cough, rash
- *Rare*: hyperkalaemia, worsening of renal function (in those with underlying renal ischaemia or severe heart failure), angioneurotic oedema, haematological toxicity (e.g. neutropenia, agranulocytosis)

Contraindications
- Renal vascular disease (e.g. renal artery stenosis)
- Pregnancy

Interactions
- *Diuretics*: pronounced hypotension is more likely if ramipril is used in conjunction with diuretics
- *NSAIDs*: these increase the risk of renal impairment
- *Potassium-sparing diuretics*: concomitant use of ramipril and potassium-sparing diuretics increases the risk of hyperkalaemia, especially in patients with renal impairment

Route of administration
- Oral

Note
- Microalbuminuria is an early sign of nephropathy in diabetics. There is evidence that once this is detected, ACE inhibitors reduce the risk of further renal deterioration.
- Patients should be advised to take the first dose just before bedtime to prevent first-dose hypotension.
- ACE inhibitors improve exercise tolerance and symptoms in heart failure. They also prolong life expectancy in these patients.

Related drugs
- Captopril, enalapril, fosinopril, lisinopril, perindopril, quinapril, trandolapril

Sildenafil

Class: Phosphodiesterase type 5 (PDE$_5$) inhibitor

Indications
- Male erectile dysfunction

Mechanism of action
- Penile erection in a healthy male involves nitric oxide release within the corpi cavernosa in response to sexual stimulation. Nitric oxide increases the levels of cGMP through activation of guanylate cyclase. This leads to relaxation of smooth muscle within the corpi cavernosa and allows influx of blood.
- The role of PDE$_5$ is to degrade cGMP within the corpus cavernosum. Sildenafil selectively inhibits this enzyme and hence produces erection (in response to sexual stimulation).

Adverse effects
- *Common*: headache, flushing, nasal congestion, dyspepsia, visual disturbance
- *Rare*: cardiovascular events, priapism, dizziness, hypersensitivity

Contraindications
- Concomitant use of nitrates
- Hypotension
- Recent stroke
- MI and unstable angina
- Hereditary degenerative disorders of the retina

Interactions
- *Nicorandil*: concomitant use may lead to profound hypotension
- *Nitrates*: concomitant use may lead to profound hypotension
- *Ritonavir*: this raises the plasma concentration of sildenafil

Route of administration
- Oral

Note
- At recommended doses sildenafil will not produce an erection without sexual stimulation.
- It is effective in roughly 70% of patients.
- After taking a dose of sildenafil, the patient has a 4 h window to engage in sexual intercourse. Other PDE$_5$ inhibitors have a longer duration of action (16 h for vardenafil, 3 days for tadalafil).

Related drugs
- Tadalafil, vardenafil

Simvastatin

Class: HMG CoA reductase inhibitor

Indications
- Hypercholesterolaemia
- Mixed hyperlipidaemia

Mechanism of action
- Simvastatin reversibly inhibits HMG CoA reductase, the rate-limiting enzyme in cholesterol synthesis by the liver. The liver responds by increasing expression of LDL receptors, which increases LDL uptake from the plasma. These actions reduce plasma cholesterol.
- Simvastatin causes a small decrease in the plasma concentration of triglycerides.

Adverse effects
- *Common*: headache, muscle cramps, flatulence
- *Rare*: reversible myositis, GI disturbance (diarrhoea, abdominal pain), rash, alopecia, altered LFTs, hepatitis, pancreatitis

Contraindications
- Liver disease
- Pregnancy and breastfeeding
- Porphyria

Interactions
- *Erythromycin and clarithromycin*: these increase the risk of myositis if given with simvastatin
- *Fibrates*: these increase the risk of myositis if given with simvastatin
- *Itraconazole and ketoconazole*: these increase the risk of myopathy if given with simvastatin
- *Warfarin*: simvastatin enhances the effect of warfarin

Route of administration
- Oral

Note
- Simvastatin has been shown to be effective in reducing cardiovascular events and mortality in patients with known, or at high risk of, cardiovascular disease.
- Simvastatin should only be prescribed if the patient has not responded sufficiently to diet modification and after secondary causes of hyperlipidaemia have been ruled out (e.g. hypothyroidism, chronic alcohol abuse).
- LFTs should be carried out before and 3 months after starting therapy and regularly thereafter.
- The patient should be advised to immediately report unexplained muscle pain, tenderness or weakness.

Related drugs
- Atorvastatin, fluvastatin, pravastatin, rosuvastatin

Tenecteplase

Class: Fibrinolytic agent

Indications
- Acute myocardial infarction

Mechanism of action
- Tenecteplase is a tissue plasminogen activator (tPA).
- It binds to circulating plasminogen in the blood and forms an activator complex that converts plasminogen to plasmin. Plasmin then lyses the fibrin within the thrombus, thus dissolving it.

Adverse effects
- *Common*: bleeding from vascular puncture sites, GI bleed from occult peptic ulcers, nausea, vomiting, hypotension
- *Rare*: intracerebral haemorrhage, allergic reaction

Contraindications
- Recent haemorrhage
- Bleeding disorders
- Recent trauma or surgery
- Aortic dissection
- Severe hepatic impairment
- Acute pancreatitis
- Coma
- Severe hypertension
- Suspected peptic ulcer

Interactions
- *Warfarin*: this increases the risk of haemorrhage if given with fibrinolytic agents

Route of administration
- IV

Note
- Fresh frozen plasma with tranexamic acid (an antifibrinolytic agent) may be given if treatment results in excessive bleeding.
- Thrombolysis with tenecteplase or reteplase is becoming the preferred option in acute MI; however, streptokinase is still commonly used as it is cost-saving.
- Alteplase and streptokinase can be used in PE. Streptokinase can also be used in DVT, acute arterial thromboembolism, thrombosed arteriovenous shunts and central retinal venous or arterial thrombosis.
- Tenecteplase, alteplase or reteplase are preferred over streptokinase if the patient presents within 6 h of onset of chest pain with evidence of anterior infarction. They are also used if the patient has had streptokinase in the past.

Related drugs
- Alteplase (rt-PA), reteplase, streptokinase

Verapamil

Class: Calcium channel blocker

Indications
- Hypertension
- Angina
- Supraventricular dysrhythmias

Mechanism of action
- Verapamil inhibits influx of calcium into vascular smooth muscle and myocardium by binding to the L-type calcium channels. This results in:

  1 Relaxation of vascular smooth muscle with subsequent decrease in peripheral resistance and blood pressure;

  2 Decreased myocardial contractility; and

  3 Slowed conduction through the AV node and prolonged refractory period (antiarrhythmic properties).
- Angina is relieved by reduction in afterload, heart rate and myocardial contractility.

Adverse effects
- *Common*: constipation, headache, ankle swelling
- *Rare*: cardiac failure, hypotension, AV node block

Contraindications
- Heart failure/cardiogenic shock
- Hypotension
- Myocardial conduction defects (e.g. bradycardia, AV node block)
- Porphyria

Interactions
- *Amiodarone*: concomitant use of amiodarone and verapamil increases the risk of AV block, bradycardia and myocardial depression
- *Beta blockers*: if beta blockers are given with or prior to verapamil there is an increased risk of AV node block, which may be complete and result in asystole, heart failure and severe hypotension
- *Digoxin*: verapamil increases the plasma concentration

Route of administration
- IV (only in paroxysmal tachydysrhythmias), oral

Note
- Beta blockers are the preferred treatment in unstable angina as they have been shown to reduce the associated risk of MI. However, if beta blockers are ineffective, verapamil can be used.

Related drugs
- Diltiazem

Warfarin

Class: Oral anticoagulant (vitamin K antagonist)

Indications
- Prevention of thromboembolism (e.g. in atrial fibrillation, prosthetic heart valves)
- Treatment and prevention of DVT and PE
- Prevention of transient ischaemic attacks and CVAs

Mechanism of action
- Vitamin K is an essential cofactor for synthesis of clotting factors II, VII, IX and X, and proteins C and S. Warfarin inhibits reduction of vitamin K by inhibiting the enzyme vitamin K epoxide reductase, thereby reducing production of the clotting factors.
- Warfarin takes at least 48–72 h to achieve its full anticoagulant effect (this reflects the half-life of the clotting factors).

Adverse effects
- *Common*: haemorrhage
- *Rare*: skin necrosis, liver damage, alopecia, pancreatitis, diarrhoea, nausea, vomiting, rash

Contraindications
- Pregnancy
- Severe hypertension
- Active peptic ulcer disease
- Bacterial endocarditis

Interactions
- *Alcohol, amiodarone, cimetidine, omeprazole and simvastatin*: these drugs increase the anticoagulant effect of warfarin
- *Aspirin, clopidogrel*: increased risk of haemorrhage
- *Carbamazepine, rifampicin*: these decrease the anticoagulant effect of warfarin
- *COC pill*: decreased anticoagulant effect
- *Note*: Warfarin is metabolised by hepatic enzymes that can be induced or inhibited by other drugs; hence a wide range of further interactions exists

Route of administration
- Oral

Note
- Therapy should be assessed regularly by measuring INR. The target INR varies with different conditions.
- Warfarin may rarely cause fetal abnormalities if taken during pregnancy (e.g. chondrodysplasia punctata).
- In severe haemorrhage warfarin should be stopped and IV vitamin K with clotting factors II, VII, IX and X should be given. If clotting factors are unavailable, fresh frozen plasma can be used.

Related drugs
- Nicoumalone, phenindione

Management guidelines (pp. 39–41)
Asthma
  Acute
  Chronic
Chronic obstructive pulmonary disease

Individual drugs (pp. 42–48)
Beclometasone; Ipratropium; Montelukast; Oxygen;
Salbutamol; Sodium cromoglicate; Theophylline

ACUTE ASTHMA
Treatment must not be delayed for investigations
• Therapy is guided by clinical state (e.g. heart rate, respiratory
rate, ability to complete sentences, BP) and peak expiratory
flow rate
• Give high-flow oxygen through face mask
• Give nebulised salbutamol via an oxygen-driven nebuliser
• Give IV hydrocortisone or oral prednisolone
• Perform ABGs if there are life-threatening features: PEF
$< 33\%$ of best or predicted, oxygen saturation $< 92\%$, silent
chest, feeble respiratory effort, bradycardia, dysrhythmia,
exhaustion, hypotension, confusion, coma
• Perform a CXR to exclude other conditions (e.g.
pneumothorax)
• Check response to treatment by monitoring oxygen
saturation, measuring peak expiratory flow rate and repeating
ABGs
• If the patient fails to respond to treatment or is deteriorating
(e.g. decreasing peak expiratory flow rate):
  • Add ipratropium bromide to the salbutamol nebuliser and
  administer nebulised beta 2 agonist more frequently (e.g.
  salbutamol up to every 15 min)
  • Consider administering a single dose of magnesium
  sulphate IV
  • If no improvement, discuss with senior clinician and ITU
  team and consider IV aminophylline (loading dose is
  contraindicated if taking oral theophylline) or IV
  salbutamol
  • If, despite this, the patient fails to improve (especially if
  P_{CO_2} is rising), consider transfer to ITU and mechanical
  ventilation
• If the patient is improving, conduct the following until
stabilised:
  • Give oxygen and 4-hourly nebulised salbutamol
  • Give daily oral prednisolone or 6-hourly IV
  hydrocortisone

- Before discharge from hospital consider stepping up usual treatment (see Chronic Asthma), educating about compliance and checking inhaler technique
- *Note*: Leukotriene antagonists are currently not recommended in the management of acute asthma

CHRONIC ASTHMA

- Educate and avoid sensitising factors (e.g. pollen, cats, beta blockers)
- Start therapy at step 1 and proceed to the next step if treatment fails to control symptoms:
  - Step 1: Inhaled beta 2 agonist (e.g. salbutamol) as required
  - Step 2: Add regular low dose inhaled corticosteroid (e.g. beclometasone)
  - Step 3: Add regular inhaled LABA. Continue if good response. If benefit is seen but control still inadequate, continue LABA and increase inhaled corticosteroid dose. If no response to LABA, stop it and increase inhaled corticosteroid dose.
  - Step 4: Consider trials of:
    1 Oral leukotriene antagonist (e.g. montelukast)
    2 Maximum dose inhaled corticosteroids
    3 Oral theophylline
    4 Oral beta 2 agonist
  - Step 5: Add regular oral corticosteroid (prednisolone), maximise other treatments and refer for specialist care
- Review treatment every 3–6 months

CHRONIC OBSTRUCTIVE PULMONARY DISEASE (COPD)

- Advise to stop smoking
- Spirometry is essential to make an accurate diagnosis, to assess disease severity and to monitor progression
- If significant reversible obstruction is present, treat as asthma
- **Use of inhaled corticosteroids in COPD**
  - Inhaled corticosteroids should only be used where objective benefit was shown in a therapeutic trial, in patients with $FEV_1 < 50\%$ predicted, or in patients with frequent exacerbations
  - Inhaled corticosteroids do not slow the decline in lung function or decrease the mortality from COPD
  - Inhaled corticosteroids may reduce the frequency of exacerbations
  - Inhaled corticosteroids are prescribed to $> 75\%$ of patients with moderate to severe COPD
- **Acute hospital admission with COPD**
  - Regular nebulised bronchodilators (e.g. salbutamol)
  - Measure ABGs:
    - If hypoxia is present, administer up to 28% oxygen with repeated blood gases

- If hypercapnia is present, discuss with respiratory physician as ventilatory support may be required
- For infective acute exacerbations, add appropriate antibiotics. If baseline $FEV_1 < 50\%$ predicted, add prednisolone for 10 days.
- Chest physiotherapy to prevent accumulation of secretions
- **COPD in the community:**
  - Diuretics for any associated cor pulmonale (right-sided heart failure secondary to chronic lung disease)
  - Long-term oxygen therapy if $P_{O_2} < 7.3\,\text{kPa}$ on more than one occasion when clinically stable
  - Influenza vaccine should be offered

Beclometasone

Class: Corticosteroid

Indications
- Prophylaxis of asthma
- Inflammatory skin disorders (e.g. eczema, psoriasis)
- Prophylaxis and treatment of allergic or vasomotor rhinitis

Mechanism of action
- Beclometasone indirectly inhibits the formation of inflammatory mediators (e.g. prostaglandins, leukotrienes), thus decreasing inflammation.
- In asthma it acts by reducing airway inflammation, which leads to decreased oedema and decreased mucous secretion.

Adverse effects
- *Common*: cough and oral candidiasis (with inhaled route), nasal irritation (with nasal spray), thinning of the skin (with topical treatment)
- *Rare*: hoarse voice (with inhaled route); depigmentation, nose bleeds, disturbance of smell (with long-term nasal spray); acne at the site of application (with topical treatment); glaucoma, cataract

Contraindications
- Skin ointment is contraindicated in acne vulgaris, rosacea and skin infections
- Nasal spray is contraindicated in untreated nasal infections and after nasal surgery until healing is complete

Interactions
- *Antiepileptics*: metabolism of beclometasone is accelerated by carbamazepine and phenytoin

Route of administration
- Inhalation (asthma), topical (skin conditions), nasal spray (rhinitis)

Note
- Using a spacer with the inhaler can prevent oral candidiasis and hoarseness. Additionally, the mouth can be rinsed out with water after using the inhaler.
- The issue of high-dose inhaled steroids and systemic adverse effects remains controversial. Some systemic absorption does occur, even with the inhaled route.
- As beclometasone reduces bone mineral density, long-term use may predispose to osteoporosis.
- Growth should be monitored in children on long-term treatment, as corticosteroids may cause growth retardation. This is much less likely with inhaled therapy than with oral corticosteroids.
- Patients with COPD usually show little or no response to inhaled beclometasone. This can help distinguish asthma from COPD.

Ipratropium

Class: Muscarinic antagonist

Indications
- COPD
- Asthma (acute and chronic)
- Rhinorrhoea

Mechanism of action
- Ipratropium is a muscarinic antagonist. It inhibits vagally mediated reflexes by antagonising the effects of acetylcholine, and thus leads to bronchodilatation and a reduction in bronchial mucous secretion.
- When applied as a nasal spray, ipratropium inhibits secretions from seromucus glands lining the nasal mucosa.

Adverse effects
- *Rare*: antimuscarinic effects (e.g. urinary retention, dry mouth), glaucoma (with nebulised route)

Contraindications
- None
- Caution:
  - Glaucoma
  - Pregnancy and breastfeeding
  - Bladder outflow obstruction
  - Prostatic hyperplasia

Interactions
- No significant interactions

Route of administration
- Inhalation (aerosol, powder, nebulised solution), nasal spray

Note
- Ipratropium is a polar molecule that is poorly absorbed and thus has very few systemic effects. However, if administered via a nebuliser, it can cause glaucoma through direct topical effect on the eyes.
- Ipratropium is thought to be more effective in relieving bronchoconstriction in COPD than in asthma.

Related drugs
- Oxitropium, tiotropium

Montelukast

Class: Leukotriene receptor antagonist

Indications
- Prophylaxis of asthma
- Treatment of chronic asthma

Mechanism of action
- Montelukast is a selective, competitive antagonist at cysteinyl leukotriene receptors. Cysteinyl leukotrienes are products of arachidonic acid metabolism. They have been implicated in the pathophysiological processes of asthma and are known to be very potent bronchoconstrictors.

Adverse effects
- *Common*: headache, rash, dizziness, dyspepsia, abdominal pain
- *Rare*: anaphylaxis, sleep disorders, palpitations

Contraindications
- None
- Caution:
  - Churg–Strauss syndrome
  - Pregnancy
  - Breastfeeding

Interactions
- *Phenobarbital*: this reduces the plasma concentration of montelukast

Route of administration
- Oral

Note
- Montelukast is no more effective than inhaled corticosteroids in the management of chronic asthma. When used together, however, these two drugs have an additive effect.
- Montelukast should not be used in the management of acute asthma.
- The use of montelukast has been associated with Churg–Strauss syndrome.
- It is extensively metabolised by hepatic cytochrome P450 enzymes.

Related drugs
- Zafirlukast

Oxygen

Class: Therapeutic gas

Indications
- Resuscitation (up to 100% oxygen)
- High concentrations (up to 100% oxygen) for acute hypoxic events (e.g. MI, acute asthma, acute poisoning, PE)
- Low concentrations (up to 28% oxygen) in patients with respiratory disease with CO_2 retention (e.g. COPD)

Mechanism of action
- Oxygen specifically binds to haemoglobin and also dissolves in plasma. It is then transported to tissues, where it promotes aerobic respiration.
- In hypoxaemic patients oxygen decreases the work of breathing needed to maintain arterial oxygen saturation.

Adverse effects
- *Rare*: retinopathy in neonates (with high concentrations), respiratory arrest in COPD, pulmonary oedema

Contraindications
- None

Interactions
- None known

Route of administration
- Nasal cannulae, face mask, tent, hood, endotracheal tube

Note
- A humidifier should be used when oxygen is administered in high concentrations, as it can cause retrosternal discomfort and dry cough. 100% oxygen becomes uncomfortable after approximately 12 h of continuous administration, while 50% oxygen is usually safe for any period of time.
- Different face masks deliver different concentrations of oxygen: Venturi mask delivers 25–60%; Hudson mask up to 40%; Hudson mask with reservoir bag up to 80%; nasal cannulae up to 35%. Anaesthetic circuit via endotracheal tube can deliver up to 100% oxygen. Endotracheal tube is the only definite means of delivering known concentrations of oxygen.
- Oxygen should only be prescribed for home use after thorough evaluation by respiratory physicians in hospital. Patients using home oxygen should be advised of fire risks.
- Long-term home oxygen may prolong survival in patients with severe COPD and coexisting cor pulmonale (at least 15 h of oxygen should be used per day).

Salbutamol

Class: Beta 2 agonist

Indications
- Asthma
- COPD with reversible component
- Premature labour

Mechanism of action
- Salbutamol stimulates beta 2 adrenoceptors in the airways, thus generating intracellular cyclic AMP. This decreases intracellular calcium and produces bronchodilatation (as calcium is required for bronchial smooth muscle contraction).
- Increased cyclic AMP also prevents degranulation of mast cells.
- When used in premature labour, salbutamol acts by inhibiting uterine smooth muscle contraction.

Adverse effects
- *Common*: tremor, tachycardia
- *Rare*: headache, palpitations, hypokalaemia, muscle cramps, insomnia (these adverse effects are dose-dependent and therefore more common with high doses)

Contraindications
- None

Interactions
- *Corticosteroids*: high doses of corticosteroids given with high doses of salbutamol increase the risk of hypokalaemia
- *Diuretics*: high doses of salbutamol increase the risk of hypokalaemia if given with loop or thiazide diuretics
- *Theophylline*: high doses of salbutamol increase the risk of hypokalaemia if given with theophylline

Route of administration
- Asthma: inhalation (aerosol, powder, nebulised solution), IM, IV, oral
- COPD: inhalation
- Premature labour: IM or IV

Note
- Plasma potassium needs to be monitored if salbutamol is given in severe asthma. This is due to the increased risk of hypokalaemia caused by high doses of salbutamol, hypoxia and concomitant treatment with diuretics and theophylline.
- Metered-dose inhalers are only useful in patients over 8 years of age. If younger, a spacer should be used to administer inhaled salbutamol.

Related drugs
- Short-acting beta 2 antagonists: bambuterol, fenoterol, reproterol, terbutaline, tulobuterol
- LABAs: formoterol, salmeterol

Sodium cromoglicate

Class: Mast cell stabiliser

Indications
- Prophylaxis of asthma
- Allergic rhinitis
- Allergic conjunctivitis
- Food allergy

Mechanism of action
- Exact mechanism is not fully understood.
- Sodium cromoglicate may reduce calcium influx into mast cells, thus rendering them more stable, i.e. less likely to release inflammatory mediators. This occurs in the bronchial tree, the nose and the eyes.

Adverse effects
- *Common*: cough, throat irritation, stinging of the eyes (with eye drops)
- *Rare*: nausea, vomiting, joint pain, rash (all with oral administration); transient bronchospasm (with inhaled route)

Contraindications
- None

Interactions
- None known

Route of administration
- Asthma: inhalation (aerosol, powder or nebulised solution)
- Food allergy: oral
- Allergic rhinitis: nasal spray
- Allergic conjunctivitis: eye drops

Note
- Sodium cromoglicate is not used in acute exacerbations of asthma.
- Roughly one-third of patients taking sodium cromoglicate, especially children, benefit from it.
- Sodium cromoglicate is generally less effective than inhaled corticosteroids in the prophylaxis of asthma in adults. It is therefore not commonly used in adult asthma.
- It is useful in the prevention of exercise-induced asthma.
- If transient bronchospasm is a problematic adverse effect, a beta 2 agonist can be inhaled a few minutes before sodium cromoglicate.
- Throat irritation can be avoided by rinsing the mouth with water after inhalation.

Related drugs
- Nedocromil sodium

Theophylline

Class: Methylxanthine

Indications
- Asthma

Mechanism of action
- Bronchodilatation is thought to be achieved by a variety of mechanisms, including inhibition of the enzyme phosphodiesterase, which degrades cyclic AMP. The raised cyclic AMP levels subsequently decrease intracellular calcium, resulting in bronchodilatation.
- Theophylline also blocks adenosine receptors, which results in smooth muscle relaxation in the bronchi.
- It increases the force of contraction of the diaphragm, possibly by enhancing calcium uptake.
- Theophylline is further believed to inhibit inflammatory cells such as mast cells.

Adverse effects
- *Common*: nausea, vomiting, headache, palpitations, tachycardia
- *Rare*: hypokalaemia, diarrhoea, CNS stimulation (insomnia, irritability, fine tremor), convulsions, dysrhythmias

Contraindications
- None
- Caution:
  - Cardiac disease (risk of dysrhythmias)
  - Hypertension
  - Epilepsy

Interactions
- *Ciprofloxacin*: this increases the plasma concentration of theophylline
- *Diltiazem, verapamil*: these increase the plasma concentration of theophylline
- *Erythromycin*: this increases the plasma concentration of theophylline
- *Note*: Theophylline is metabolised by hepatic enzymes that can be induced or inhibited by other drugs; hence a wide range of further interactions exists

Route of administration
- IV (as aminophylline, in acute severe asthma), oral

Note
- Therapeutic drug monitoring is recommended.
- Oral sustained-release tablets are available, which are effective for up to 12 h (less adverse effects).
- Theophylline can be given in combination with ethylene-diamine as aminophylline. This is more readily absorbed and has fewer GI adverse effects.
- Theophylline and aminophylline should not be given together due to the risk of serious adverse effects (e.g. convulsions or dysrhythmias).

Related drugs
- Aminophylline

GASTROINTESTINAL SYSTEM

Management guidelines (pp. 49–51)
Constipation
Crohn's disease
Diarrhoea
Helicobacter pylori infection
Peptic ulcer disease
Ulcerative colitis

Individual drugs (pp. 52–65)
Antacids; Cyclizine; Ferrous sulphate; Folic acid;
Hydroxocobalamin; Lactulose; Loperamide; Metoclopramide;
Omeprazole; Ondansetron; Pancreatin; Ranitidine; Senna;
Sulfasalazine

CONSTIPATION
• Treat any underlying cause
• Recommend high-fibre diet with adequate fluid intake
• If the above fails, consider any of the following laxatives:
• Bulking agents (e.g. bran, ispaghula husk, methylcellulose)
• Osmotic laxatives (e.g. lactulose, macrogols, magnesium salts)
• Stimulant laxatives (e.g. bisacodyl, senna, docusate sodium, dantron)
• Stool softeners (rarely used, e.g. arachis oil)

CROHN'S DISEASE
• **In mild to moderate disease:**
  • Administer a 5-ASA preparation (e.g. sulfasalazine, mesalazine)
  • If no improvement, consider adding metronidazole or ciprofloxacin
  • If still no improvement, treat as moderate to severe disease
• **In moderate to severe disease:**
  • Administer systemic steroids (e.g. prednisolone or budesonide) until symptoms resolve. Not to be used for maintenance due to adverse effects.
  • Consider parenteral nutrition (allows bowel rest)
  • If no improvement with above therapy, consider starting infliximab (monoclonal antibody that inhibits tumour necrosis factor α)
• *Note*:
  • Surgery may be required for bowel obstruction, perforation, perianal disease, haemorrhage or fistula formation

- Consider adding immunosuppressants (e.g. azathioprine) as maintenance if other measures fail. It may take up to 4 months before any benefit is seen.

DIARRHOEA
- Remember that most cases of diarrhoea are self-limiting and often caused by viruses (e.g. rotavirus)
- Antibiotics are not usually required for simple gastroenteritis
- Aim of treatment is to replace fluid and electrolyte losses by oral rehydration therapy (IV in nausea and vomiting)
- The following can be given for symptomatic relief in uncomplicated acute diarrhoea in adults (but rule out infectious diarrhoea with stool samples first):
  - Loperamide
  - Codeine phosphate
  - Diphenoxylate
  - *Note*: Antimotility agents should not be used in the management of acute diarrhoea in children
- Common bacterial causes of diarrhoea are *Campylobacter*, *Shigella* and *Giardia* spp. See p. 129 for treatment.
- Investigate with sigmoidoscopy or colonoscopy if diarrhoea persists for longer than 6 weeks

HELICOBACTER PYLORI INFECTION
- Confirm the presence of *H. pylori* prior to starting eradication treatment (e.g. serology, ^{13}C-urea breath test)
- Triple therapy (proton pump inhibitor + amoxicillin + *either* metronidazole *or* clarithromycin) for 1 week eradicates *H. pylori* in > 90% of cases
- Treatment failure is usually due to poor compliance or antibacterial resistance

PEPTIC ULCER DISEASE
- Most gastric ulcers (70–75%) and nearly all duodenal ulcers (90–100%) are caused by *H. pylori* infection. The rest are due to NSAIDs.
- Stop NSAIDs (if appropriate)
- Reduce exacerbating factors (e.g. smoking, obesity, alcohol, spicy foods). These measures, however, have been less important since the discovery of *H. pylori*.
- Administer triple therapy for *H. pylori* infection (if appropriate)
- A proton pump inhibitor (e.g. omeprazole) given for 4 weeks should heal 90% of duodenal ulcers; it should also heal 80–90% of gastric ulcers if given for 8 weeks
- H_2 antagonists (e.g. ranitidine) are less effective than proton pump inhibitors and are not commonly used for the treatment of peptic ulcers

- Other medical treatment options include ulcer-healing agents (e.g. bismuth, sucralfate)
- In resistant cases consider surgery (e.g. vagotomy $+/-$ pyloroplasty for a duodenal ulcer; partial gastrectomy for a gastric ulcer)

ULCERATIVE COLITIS

- Give a 5-ASA preparation as maintenance therapy (e.g. sulfasalazine, mesalazine)
- Administer rectal 5-ASA for acute proctitis and proctosigmoiditis
- Administer systemic 5 ASA for more extensive disease
- Add systemic corticosteroids (e.g. prednisolone) in severe acute ulcerative colitis, or in moderate colitis not responding to maximum dose of 5-ASA.
- If still no improvement after 5 days of therapy, consider IV ciclosporin
- If still no improvement, consider surgery
- *Note*: There is no evidence to suggest that antibiotics are useful in the management of ulcerative colitis

Antacids

(Aluminium salts, magnesium salts, sodium bicarbonate)

Indications
- Symptomatic relief of:
  - Ulcer dyspepsia
  - Gastro-oesophageal reflux disease
  - Severe metabolic acidosis (sodium bicarbonate)
  - Alkalinisation of urine (sodium bicarbonate)

Mechanism of action
- Antacids are weak alkalis that neutralise the acid in the stomach.

Adverse effects
- *Common*: constipation (aluminium salts), diarrhoea (magnesium salts), belching (sodium bicarbonate)
- *Rare*: metabolic alkalosis

Contraindications
- Hypophosphataemia (aluminium and magnesium salts)
- Caution:
  - Salt restriction diet (sodium bicarbonate)
  - Renal impairment (magnesium salts)

Interactions
- *ACE inhibitors, antibacterials, digoxin, iron*: antacids decrease the absorption of these drugs
- *Lithium*: sodium bicarbonate increases the excretion of lithium

Route of administration
- Oral

Note
- Some antacids are combined with alginates to further suppress acid reflux. Alginates protect the oesophagus by forming a 'raft', which decreases acid regurgitation.
- Most antacids are not absorbed from the GI tract and therefore rarely cause systemic adverse effects.
- Dimeticone (antifoaming agent) can be added to antacids to reduce flatulence.
- In UTIs, sodium bicarbonate can alkalinise the urine. This relieves dysuria.
- Sodium bicarbonate may also be used in the form of ear drops to soften ear wax.
- Benefit of antacids in the management of non-ulcer dyspepsia is uncertain.
- Preparations containing more than one antacid do not have a superior effect in comparison to simple preparations.

Cyclizine

Class: Histamine 1 receptor antagonist

Indications
- Nausea and vomiting
- Labyrinthine disturbances and vertigo
- Motion sickness

Mechanism of action
- Cyclizine acts as a competitive antagonist at histamine 1 receptors in the vomiting centre of the brain.
- It also has weak antimuscarinic effects and is mildly sedating.

Adverse effects
- *Common*: headache
- *Rare*: insomnia, palpitations, antimuscarinic effects (e.g. urinary retention, dry mouth), drowsiness

Contraindications
- Porphyria
- Caution:
  - Hepatic disease
  - Urinary retention and prostatic hypertrophy

Interactions
- *Alcohol*: this enhances the sedative effect of cyclizine
- *Antimuscarinics*: these enhance the antimuscarinic adverse effects of cyclizine

Route of administration
- Oral, IM, IV

Note
- Antiemetics should only be administered when the cause of nausea is known, as they may otherwise delay diagnosis.
- A combination of two antiemetics with different sites of action may be effective in nausea and vomiting that is not alleviated by a single agent.
- Unlike metoclopramide, cyclizine is effective in the treatment of motion sickness.
- Cyclizine is a safe antiemetic in pregnancy.

Related drugs
- Cinnarizine, meclozine, promethazine

Ferrous sulphate

Class: Iron salt

Indications
- Iron-deficiency anaemia

Mechanism of action
- Ferrous sulphate replenishes iron stores.

Adverse effects
- *Common*: nausea, epigastric pain, constipation or diarrhoea, darkening of faeces (often confused with melaena)

Contraindications
- None
- Caution:
  - Pregnancy

Interactions
- *Magnesium salts*: these reduce the absorption of iron
- *Quinolone anitbiotics*: iron reduces absorption of these drugs
- *Tetracycline*: absorption of ferrous sulphate is decreased by tetracycline

Route of administration
- Oral

Note
- The cause of iron-deficiency anaemia should be sought prior to administration of ferrous sulphate.
- Iron deficiency causes hypochromic microcytic anaemia with low serum ferritin levels and increased TIBC.
- Hb concentration increases by roughly 2 g/100 ml with every 3–4 weeks of treatment.
- In order to replenish iron stores, treatment with oral ferrous sulphate is continued for 3–6 months after Hb levels have reached the normal range.
- Patients unable to tolerate oral iron (e.g. because of severe adverse effects) should be given iron sorbitol by deep IM injection.
- Absorption of ferrous sulphate can be improved by combining it with vitamin C.
- Potentially fatal iron poisoning (nausea, vomiting, bloody diarrhoea, haematemesis, abdominal pain, hypotension and coma) is commonest in children.

Related drugs
- Ferrous fumarate, ferrous gluconate

Folic acid

Class: Vitamin supplement

Indications
- Prevention of neural tube defects in pregnancy
- Folate-deficient megaloblastic anaemia
- End-stage renal failure
- Chronic haemolytic states
- Prevention of folate deficiency in patients taking anticonvulsants (phenytoin, carbamazepine)

Mechanism of action
- Folic acid has a role in cell metabolism due to its ability to transfer single carbon atom–containing groups. This is important in the synthesis of purines and pyrimidines and therefore in the synthesis of DNA.

Adverse effects
- None

Contraindications
- Folic acid alone should not be given to patients with anaemia secondary to vitamin B_{12} deficiency as this may precipitate subacute combined degeneration of the spinal cord. In this case it should be administered in conjunction with vitamin B_{12}.

Interactions
- No significant interactions

Route of administration
- Oral

Note
- The cause of folate deficiency should be ascertained and corrected prior to folate therapy.
- Folate is absorbed in the proximal jejunum. Folate deficiency is therefore a leading finding in coeliac disease.
- In order to prevent fetal neural tube defects, women should be started on daily folic acid supplements prior to conception and should continue until the 12th week of pregnancy.

Hydroxocobalamin

Class: Vitamin B_{12}

Indications
- Pernicious anaemia
- Other vitamin B_{12}–deficiency states (e.g. following gastrectomy or total ileal resection)
- Leber's optic atrophy
- Schilling test

Mechanism of action
- Hydroxocobalamin is needed for synthesis of purines and pyrimidines and their subsequent incorporation into DNA.

Adverse effects
- *Rare*: anaphylaxis, nausea, dizziness, pruritus, fever

Contraindications
- None

Interactions
- None

Route of administration
- IM

Note
- Hydroxocobalamin has replaced cyanocobalamin as therapeutic vitamin B_{12} because it is retained in the body for a longer period of time.
- Dietary vitamin B_{12} is absorbed in the terminal ileum.
- Schilling test is employed in the diagnosis of pernicious anaemia.
- Hydroxocobalamin injections are given on alternate days for the first few weeks and once every 3 months thereafter as maintenance therapy (usually for life).

Lactulose

Class: Osmotic laxative

Indications
- Constipation
- Hepatic encephalopathy

Mechanism of action
- Lactulose is a disaccharide consisting of fructose and galactose.
- Lactulose stimulates bowel peristalsis by increasing the volume of intestinal contents. It cannot be metabolised by human disaccharidases, and reaches the colon virtually unchanged, where it is hydrolysed by bacteria into simple organic acids (mainly lactic acid). These components draw water into the lumen of the large bowel by osmosis.
- Lactulose also decreases pH of the gut contents, thus reducing the activity of ammonia-producing organisms. Hence its use in hepatic encephalopathy (ammonia is thought to cross the blood–brain barrier and act as a false neurotransmitter, thus causing the symptoms of hepatic encephalopathy).

Adverse effects
- *Common*: flatulence, abdominal cramps, diarrhoea
- *Rare*: abdominal distension

Contraindications
- Intestinal obstruction
- Galactosaemia

Interactions
- None (as it is not absorbed)

Route of administration
- Oral

Note
- Lactulose can take up to 48 h to have an effect.
- It can be given to prevent constipation caused by opioids.

Related drugs
- Macrogols, magnesium salts, phosphates, sodium citrate

Loperamide

Class: Opioid antimotility drug

Indications
- Symptomatic management of acute diarrhoea
- Supplement to rehydration in acute diarrhoea (patients over 4 years of age only)
- Chronic diarrhoea (adults only)

Mechanism of action
- Loperamide acts on opioid μ receptors in the myenteric plexus of the gut wall. It inhibits acetylcholine release from the myenteric plexus and hence inhibits peristalsis.
- It also increases the tone of the anal sphincter.

Adverse effects
- *Common*: abdominal cramps
- *Rare*: constipation, abdominal bloating, rash, paralytic ileus

Contraindications
- Active ulcerative colitis
- Antibiotic-associated colitis
- Dysentery

Interactions
- None

Route of administration
- Oral

Note
- Loperamide should not be used for long periods of time. Further investigation into the cause of diarrhoea should be undertaken if no improvement is seen after a few days of treatment.
- Unlike other opioids, loperamide does not easily penetrate the blood–brain barrier, which makes it unlikely to cause central effects and dependence.

Related drugs
- Codeine phosphate, co-phenotrope, morphine, diphenoxylate

Metoclopramide

Class: Dopamine 2 antagonist

Indications
- Nausea and vomiting (due to drugs, chemotherapy, radiotherapy, migraine)
- Gastro-oesophageal reflux
- Barium follow-through investigation

Mechanism of action
- Metoclopramide has several actions, all of which contribute to its antiemetic effect:

  1 It blocks dopamine 2 receptors in the chemoreceptor trigger zone in the brainstem.

  2 It increases the rate of gastric and duodenal emptying by causing relaxation of the pyloric sphincter. It also increases lower oesophageal sphincter tone.

- In barium follow-through, metoclopramide speeds up barium transit.

Adverse effects
- *Rare*: tardive dyskinesia, neuroleptic malignant syndrome, hyperprolactinaemia, depression, cardiac conduction abnormalities, diarrhoea, acute dystonic reactions (e.g. oculogyric crisis)

Contraindications
- Intestinal obstruction, haemorrhage or perforation
- The first 3–4 days following GI surgery
- Breastfeeding
- Phaeochromocytoma

Interactions
- *Analgesics*: metoclopramide increases the absorption of paracetamol and aspirin thus enhancing their effects
- *Antipsychotics*: metoclopramide increases the risk of extrapyramidal adverse effects

Route of administration
- Oral, IM, IV

Note
- Nausea and vomiting in migraine can cause gastric stasis, which reduces the absorption rate of aspirin and paracetamol. In order to accelerate their absorption, aspirin and paracetamol can be combined with metoclopramide.
- Acute dystonic reactions are more common in young females taking metoclopramide. These can be treated with a muscarinic antagonist (e.g. benzatropine).
- Metoclopramide is not effective against motion sickness.
- Domperidone has similar pharmacological actions to metoclopramide, but is less likely to cause CNS effects due to its poor transport across the blood–brain barrier.

Related drugs
- Domperidone

Omeprazole

Class: Proton pump inhibitor

Indications
- Prophylaxis and treatment of gastric or duodenal ulcers
- Part of *H. pylori* eradication therapy
- Gastro-oesophageal reflux/oesophagitis
- Zollinger–Ellison syndrome

Mechanism of action
- Omeprazole causes dose-dependent irreversible inhibition of gastric acid production by inhibiting the H^+/K^+ ATPase ('proton pump') in gastric parietal cells. Acid secretion is thus inhibited by over 90%.
- Omeprazole is activated at a pH of less than 3.

Adverse effects
- *Common*: headache, diarrhoea, constipation
- *Rare*: Stevens–Johnson syndrome, gynaecomastia, hypersensitivity reactions, hepatic or renal impairment, blurred vision, haematological disorders (e.g. pancytopenia, thrombocytopenia), vomiting

Contraindications
- None
- Caution:
  - Liver disease
  - Pregnancy
  - Breastfeeding

Interactions
- *Phenytoin*: omeprazole increases the plasma concentration of phenytoin
- *Warfarin*: omeprazole increases the plasma concentration of warfarin
- *Note*: Omeprazole inhibits hepatic drug-metabolising enzymes; hence a wide range of further interactions exists

Route of administration
- Oral, IV

Note
- Achlorhydria (absence of acid) is linked with gastric cancer, and for this reason some physicians are concerned about long-term therapy with proton pump inhibitors. Reduced gastric acidity may also predispose to GI infections.
- Omeprazole may also mask the symptoms of gastric cancer. It is therefore important to exclude malignancy prior to treatment.
- Omeprazole is more efficient at reducing gastric acidity and has a longer duration of action than histamine 2 antagonists. Proton pump inhibitors heal roughly 90% of duodenal ulcers after 4 weeks of therapy, and have lower recurrence rates than with histamine 2 antagonists.
- Proton pump inhibitors are considered gold standard treatment for gastric ulcers with 80–90% healing rates after 8 weeks of therapy.

Related drugs
- Esomeprazole, lansoprazole, pantoprazole, rabeprazole

Ondansetron

Class: Serotonin (5-HT$_3$) antagonist

Indications
- Treatment and prophylaxis of nausea and vomiting (in chemotherapy, radiotherapy and postoperatively)

Mechanism of action
- Exact mechanism is not fully understood.
- Ondansetron selectively blocks excitatory serotonin receptors in the chemoreceptor trigger zone of the brain and in the GI tract.

Adverse effects
- *Common*: headache, constipation, flushing
- *Rare*: deranged LFTs, transient visual disturbances, seizures

Contraindications
- None
- Caution:
  - Pregnancy
  - Breastfeeding
  - Hepatic impairment

Interactions
- None

Route of administration
- Oral, IM, IV, rectal

Note
- The effect of ondansetron can be enhanced by adding a single dose of dexamethasone for chemotherapy-induced nausea and vomiting.

Related drugs
- Granisetron, tropisetron

Pancreatin

Class: Enzyme-containing pancreas extract

Indications
- Reduced or absent pancreatic exocrine secretions (e.g. in cystic fibrosis, chronic pancreatitis, following pancreatectomy)

Mechanism of action
- Pancreatin contains protease for breakdown of proteins, amylase for breakdown of starch and lipase for breakdown of fats.
- These enzymes are essential for an efficient digestive process.

Adverse effects
- *Common*: nausea, vomiting, diarrhoea, abdominal discomfort
- *Rare*: hypersensitivity, perianal irritation (with excessive doses)

Contraindications
- None

Interactions
- No significant interactions

Route of administration
- Oral

Note
- Pancreatin should be taken with food. Additionally, histamine 2 receptor antagonists (e.g. ranitidine) or antacids can be given in conjunction with pancreatin to prevent destruction of the pancreatic enzymes by gastric acid.
- Excessive heat inactivates the enzymes contained in pancreatin. It should therefore not be mixed with hot foods or hot liquids.
- Enteric-coated preparations carry more of the enzymes to the duodenum. This makes pancreatin therapy more efficient.

Ranitidine

Class: Histamine 2 antagonist

Indications
- Gastro-oesophageal reflux disease
- Prophylaxis of NSAID-associated gastric or duodenal ulcers
- Treatment of duodenal and gastric ulcers

Mechanism of action
- Ranitidine decreases gastric acid production by roughly 80%. It does so by acting as a competitive antagonist at membrane-bound histamine 2 receptors on parietal cells in the stomach.
- Maximum therapeutic response is achieved in fasting state.

Adverse effects
- *Common*: diarrhoea, deranged LFTs, rash, dizziness
- *Rare*: acute pancreatitis, cardiac dysrhythmias, confusion, alopecia, erythema multiforme

Contraindications
- None
- Caution:
  - Porphyria

Interactions
- No significant interactions

Route of administration
- Oral, IM, IV

Note
- Ranitidine should heal roughly 90% of duodenal ulcers after 8 weeks of therapy. It can also be used to treat gastric ulcers; however, proton pump inhibitors (e.g. omeprazole) are preferred in this case as they are more effective.
- Gastric cancer must be excluded before prescribing ranitidine to elderly and middle-aged patients as it may mask the symptoms and thus delay diagnosis.
- Ranitidine is preferred to cimetidine because it has fewer adverse effects and fewer drug interactions. Unlike cimetidine it does not cause impotence in young men and does not cause confusion in the elderly.
- H_2 receptor antagonists are of no use in the management of acute upper GI haemorrhage.
- Unlike cimetidine, ranitidine is not a hepatic enzyme inhibitor.

Related drugs
- Cimetidine, famotidine, nizatidine

Senna

Class: Stimulant laxative

Indications
- Constipation

Mechanism of action
- Senna is hydrolysed by bacteria in the colon to produce irritant anthracene glycoside derivatives. These stimulate the myenteric (Auerbach's) plexus in the gut wall to increase peristalsis.

Adverse effects
- *Common*: abdominal cramps, diarrhoea
- *Rare*: hypokalaemia, colonic atony (with prolonged use)

Contraindications
- Intestinal obstruction

Interactions
- None

Route of administration
- Oral

Note
- Senna acts within 8–12 h.
- Regular use of senna can lead to tolerance and should therefore be used for short periods only.
- Patients taking senna should be warned about the dangers of continuous use (e.g. hypokalaemia, atonic colon).
- A high-fibre intake (e.g. fruit, vegetable, whole wheat) should be encouraged.

Related drugs
- Bisacodyl, dantron, docusate sodium, glycerol, sodium picosulphate

Sulfasalazine

Class: Aminosalicylate

Indications
- Treatment and maintenance of ulcerative colitis
- Active Crohn's disease
- Rheumatoid arthritis

Mechanism of action
- Sulfasalazine is split into 5-ASA and sulfapyridine (a sulphonamide) by colonic flora. The function of sulfapyridine is to carry 5-ASA to the gut. 5-ASA is an active anti-inflammatory agent whose mechanism of action in the large bowel is not yet clear.
- In rheumatoid arthritis, it is the sulfapyridine component which acts as a disease-modifying antirheumatic drug.

Adverse effects
- *Common*: nausea, abdominal discomfort, diarrhoea, lupus erythematosus–like syndrome
- *Rare*: blood dyscrasias (e.g. aplastic anaemia, leucopenia), acute pancreatitis, hepatitis, nephrotic syndrome, orange discoloration of urine, impotence, depression

Contraindications
- Salicylate hypersensitivity
- Renal impairment
- Children under the age of 2 years

Interactions
- No significant interactions

Route of administration
- Oral, rectal

Note
- As high doses of sulfasalazine are usually required, adverse effects can be minimised by increasing the dose slowly and using enteric-coated tablets. The risk of GI adverse effects can be reduced by maintaining an adequate fluid intake.
- As 5-ASA can cause blood dyscrasias, patients should be advised to report any unexplained bleeding, bruising or sore throat. If these symptoms occur, a FBC should be performed immediately. The drug should be discontinued if there is any suspicion of a blood dyscrasia.
- Close monitoring of FBC and LFTs is required during the first 3 months of therapy.
- Haematological abnormalities mostly occur within the first 3–6 months. They are reversible upon cessation of therapy.
- Newer aminosalicylates, such as balsalazide, mesalazine or olsalazine, have fewer adverse effects. This is due to the absence of the sulphonamide component, which is responsible for most of the adverse effects.

Related drugs
- Balsalazide, mesalazine, olsalazine

CENTRAL NERVOUS SYSTEM

Management guidelines (pp. 67–68)
Depression
Epilepsy
Migraine
Idiopathic Parkinson's disease

Drug classes (pp. 69–71)
Antidepressants
Benzodiazepines
Neuroleptics

Individual drugs (pp. 72–88)
Amitriptyline; Bromocriptine; Carbamazepine;
Chlorpromazine; Diazepam; Fluoxetine; Haloperidol;
Hyoscine; Levodopa; Lithium; Phenelzine; Phenytoin;
Risperidone; Sodium valproate; Sumatriptan; Temazepam;
Zopiclone

DEPRESSION
· Treat only if the patient is clinically depressed
· 1st line drug therapy: SSRI (e.g. fluoxetine) or a TCA (e.g.
amitriptyline)
· If still symptomatic, consider other antidepressants such as
venlafaxine or nefazodone
· If still no response, refer to a psychiatrist who may try the
following:
  · TCA + lithium
  · TCA + MAOI
  · MAOI
  · Electroconvulsive therapy
· Improvement is not usually seen until 2–6 weeks after starting
treatment
· Continue therapy for 4–6 months after depression has
resolved
· For rapid effect and for patients not responding to
antidepressants consider electroconvulsive therapy
· Psychotherapy and counselling are of benefit to some
patients. Cognitive behavioural therapy is equally as effective
as pharmacological treatment.

EPILEPSY
Partial seizures
· 1st line therapy: carbamazepine or sodium valproate
· 2nd line therapy: lamotrigine or phenytoin or topiramate
· Adjunctive therapy: gabapentin

Generalised seizures
- Absence seizures: sodium valproate or ethosuximide
- Tonic/clonic seizures: carbamazepine or sodium valproate or phenytoin or lamotrigine
- Myoclonic and atonic seizures: sodium valproate or clonazepam

Status epilepticus
- Give oxygen through face mask
- Give IV diazepam (rectal in children or if IV access not possible)
- If no response after 5 min, repeat diazepam
- Give IV thiamine if alcohol is thought to be involved
- Give 50 ml of 50% dextrose IV if blood glucose is low
- If still fitting, add IV phenytoin (attach cardiac monitor to detect any dysrhythmias induced by phenytoin)
- If still fitting after maximum dose of diazepam and phenytoin, consider phenobarbitone, get expert help and consider mechanical ventilation under general anaesthesia

MIGRAINE
Acute attacks
- Give paracetamol or soluble aspirin or other NSAIDs (e.g. diclofenac, ibuprofen)
- Metoclopramide can be given for associated nausea and vomiting (and also to increase the rate of absorption of aspirin and paracetamol)
- Give sumatriptan (a 5-HT_1 agonist) if the above fails. This can be given orally, as intranasal spray or subcutaneously.
- Ergotamine, an alpha agonist, is rarely used but may be tried if all else fails (contraindicated in IHD)

Prophylaxis
- Prophylaxis is given to patients who experience more than one severe migraine attack per month
- Avoid precipitating factors (mainly emotional factors, but also chocolate, cheese, alcohol, lack of sleep, oral contraceptive pill)
- The following drugs can be tried: oral pizotifen (a 5-HT_2 antagonist), oral propranolol or an oral TCA
- Sodium valproate may be tried if above measures fail

IDIOPATHIC PARKINSON'S DISEASE
Supportive treatment
- Physiotherapy may be helpful in maintaining joint and muscle mobility and ensuring independence
- Involve the occupational therapist, social worker and speech therapist

Pharmacological treatment
- Anti-Parkinsonian drugs improve quality of life by alleviating symptoms, but they do not prevent progression of the disease
- Treatment of choice: levodopa with a peripheral decarboxylase inhibitor (benserazide or carbidopa)
- Other options are:

1 Dopamine agonists
   - These are reserved for cases where levodopa is no longer effective or no longer tolerated
   - They are also used in younger patients with early Parkinson's disease
   - Dopamine agonists include ropinirole and lisuride (D_2 agonists), pramipexole (D_2 and D_3 agonist), apomorphine (D_1 and D_2 agonist) and bromocriptine (ergot derivative)

2 Antimuscarinics
   - These counteract the cholinergic excess that is believed to occur in Parkinson's disease
   - They are used in drug-induced Parkinsonism or if tremor is a prominent symptom
   - They include benzhexol, benzatropine and orphenadrine

3 Others
   - Adjuvant treatment: entacapone (a monoamine oxidase inhibitor), amantadine
   - Selegiline (MAO type B inhibitor) can be used early in the disease process or combined with levodopa
   - COMT inhibitors (e.g. polcapone) are sometimes used in late Parkinson's disease unresponsive to other drugs

4 Surgery
   - Stereotactic neurosurgery may be of use if all other measures fail

Drug classes

ANTIDEPRESSANTS
Types of antidepressants
- **Tricyclic antidepressants**:
  - Sedating: amitriptyline, clomipramine, dothiepin, doxepin, maprotiline, mianserin, rimipramine
  - Less-sedating: amoxapine, imipramine, lofepramine, nortriptyline
- **Selective serotonin reuptake inhibitors**: citalopram, fluoxetine, fluvoxamine, oxetine, paroxetine, sertraline
- **Monoamine oxidase inhibitors**:
  - Irreversible inhibitors: isocarboxazid, phenelzine, tranylcypromine (these have alerting rather than sedating properties)
  - Reversible inhibitors: moclobemide (2nd line treatment for major depression)
- **Others**: mirtazipine, nefazadone, venlafaxine

Adverse effects
• Cardiotoxic and antimuscarinic adverse effects in overdose make TCAs undesirable for use in patients at risk of taking overdoses (lofepramine is the only TCA that is safe in overdose)
• SSRIs are less sedating than TCAs and have fewer cardiotoxic and antimuscarinic effects. They are therefore preferred to TCAs in patients at risk of overdose.

Note
• SSRIs, TCAs and MAOIs are all about 80% effective
• Antidepressants should be withdrawn gradually. Sudden withdrawal may preciptate GI symptoms, insomnia, headaches or restlessness. SSRIs in particular have been associated with withdrawal symptoms (especially paroxetine).
• MAOIs are 2nd line agents after TCAs and SSRIs due to their hazardous drug and food interactions

BENZODIAZEPINES
Types of benzodiazepines
1 Short-acting: loprazolam, lorazepam, lormetazepam, midazolam, oxazepam, temazepam
2 Long-acting: alprazolam, clobazam, clonazepam, diazepam, flunitrazepam, flurazepam, nitrazepam

Indications
• Benzodiazepines are mainly used according to their duration of action
• Anxiety (diazepam)
• Insomnia (temazepam)
• Convulsions (diazepam in status epilepticus, clonazepam for prophylaxis)
• Sedation for medical procedures (midazolam)
• Alcohol withdrawal (diazepam)

Mechanism of action
• Benzodiazepines potentiate the inhibitory actions of GABA by binding to GABA receptors in the CNS

Adverse effects
• These are usually due to CNS effects: sedation, memory disturbance, blurred vision, ataxia, dysarthria, incontinence, nightmares, confusion, excessive salivation, respiratory depression
• If used for more than several weeks, benzodiazepines can lead to tolerance and psychological/physical dependence (especially short-acting benzodiazepines). Therefore treatment should not exceed 2 weeks at a time.

Withdrawing benzodiazepines after long-term treatment
• Arrange a 'contract' with the patient in order to increase compliance
• Reduce the dose by one-eighth every 2–4 weeks in order to avoid withdrawal symptoms
• Abrupt withdrawal of benzodiazepines can cause anxiety, tremor, seizures and rebound sleeplessness

NEUROLEPTICS
Types of neuroleptics
1 Typical
  • Phenothiazines: chlorpromazine, fluphenazine, pipothiazine, prochlorperazine, thioridazine, trifluoperazine
  • Butyrophenones: benperidol, droperidol, haloperidol
  • Thioxanthines: fluphenthixol
  • Others: pimozide
2 Atypical
  • Clozapine, olanzapine, quetiapine, sulpiride, risperidone, zotepine

Indications
• Psychosis
• In schizophrenia:
  • Typicals are effective for positive symptoms
  • Atypicals are effective for both negative and positive symptoms

Mechanism of action
• Exact mechanism is not fully understood.
• All neuroleptics block D_2 receptors in the brain. This is thought to be responsible for the antipsychotic effect.
• Atypicals additionally block $5\text{-}HT_2$ receptors.

Adverse effects
• Dopamine receptor blockade: Parkinsonism, depression, hyperprolactinaemia, tardive dyskinesia
• Muscarinic receptor blockade: dry mouth, blurred vision, constipation
• Alpha 1 adrenoceptor blockade: postural hypotension
• Histamine 1 receptor blockade: sedation
• A rare but serious adverse effect is neuroleptic malignant syndrome

Note
• Clozapine is associated with a risk of agranulocytosis and patients must therefore be monitored with regular blood counts
• Atypicals may be better tolerated than typical neuroleptics

Amitriptyline

Class: Tricyclic antidepressant

Indications
- Depression
- Neuralgia
- Nocturnal enuresis in children

Mechanism of action
- Amitriptyline increases serotonin and norepinephrine transmission in the CNS. It achieves this by inhibiting reuptake of these neurotransmitters from the synaptic cleft.
- Amitriptyline also blocks histamine 1, muscarinic and alpha 1 receptors, which can result in a wide range of adverse effects.

Adverse effects
- *Common*: sedation, dry mouth, blurred vision, postural hypotension, constipation
- *Rare*: convulsions, cardiac dysrhythmias, weight gain, difficulty in passing urine, precipitation of glaucoma, hyponatraemia

Contraindications
- Recent MI
- Cardiac dysrhythmias (especially heart block)

Interactions
- *Antiarrhythmics*: amitriptyline increases the risk of ventricular dysrhythmias if given with antiarrhythmics
- *Anticonvulsants*: amitriptyline antagonises the anticonvulsant effect
- *MAOIs*: danger of potentially fatal hyperthermia syndrome
- *Neuroleptics*: increased risk of ventricular dysrhythmias

Route of administration
- Oral

Note
- Amitriptyline must be taken regularly for 3–4 weeks before any improvement is likely.
- Treatment should be continued for at least 6 months to prevent recurrence of depression, even if the patient recovers earlier.
- Sedative properties of amitriptyline are useful in depression associated with insomnia.

Related drugs
- Amoxapine, clomipramine, dothiepin, doxepin, imipramine, lofepramine, nortriptyline, trimipramine

Bromocriptine

Class: Dopamine agonist

Indications
- Idiopathic Parkinson's disease
- Hyperprolactinaemia
- Acromegaly
- Cyclical benign breast disease
- Prevention and suppression of lactation

Mechanism of action
- Bromocriptine stimulates D_2 receptors in the CNS. This accounts for its use in Parkinson's disease.
- Bromocriptine is useful in hyperprolactinaemia as it inhibits the release of prolactin from the anterior pituitary gland. This inhibits lactation. Bromocriptine also reduces the size of prolactinomas.
- Bromocriptine inhibits the release of growth hormone in acromegaly (NB: in unaffected individuals growth hormone levels are raised by bromocriptine).

Adverse effects
- *Common*: nausea, vomiting, constipation, postural hypotension
- *Rare*: confusion, drowsiness, dyskinesia, vasospasm in fingers and toes, pulmonary or retroperitoneal fibrosis

Contraindications
- Pre-eclampsia
- Postpartum hypertension

Interactions
- *Erythromycin*: this increases the plasma concentration of bromocriptine, thus increasing the risk of dose-dependent adverse effects

Route of administration
- Oral

Note
- High doses of bromocriptine are normally used in the treatment of acromegaly and Parkinson's disease. This leads to a higher incidence of adverse effects.
- Nausea and vomiting can be decreased by increasing the dose of bromocriptine slowly and taking it with meals.
- Domperidone can be used to reduce the systemic adverse effects of bromocriptine. It does not reduce central adverse effects as it does not cross the blood–brain barrier.

Related drugs
- Cabergoline, quinagolide

Carbamazepine

Class: Anticonvulsant

Indications
- Generalised tonic/clonic seizures
- Partial seizures
- Trigeminal neuralgia and other chronic neurogenic pain
- Prophylaxis of bipolar disorder

Mechanism of action
- Exact mechanism is not fully understood.
- Carbamazepine is thought to:
  1 Enhance GABA-mediated inhibitory transmission in the CNS.
  2 Decrease electrical excitability of neuronal cell membranes by blocking sodium channels.

Adverse effects
- *Common*: drowsiness, blurred vision, confusion, rash
- *Rare*: agranulocytosis, thrombocytopenia, hepatic failure, acute renal failure, rash, cardiac conduction abnormalities, osteomalacia, hyponatraemia, ataxia, Stevens–Johnson syndrome

Contraindications
- Bone marrow depression
- AV node conduction abnormalities (unless pacemaker in situ)
- Porphyria

Interactions
- *Diltiazem, verapamil*: these drugs increase the plasma concentration of carbamazepine
- *Oral contraceptive pill*: carbamazepine reduces the effect of oral contraceptives
- *Warfarin*: carbamazepine reduces the effect of warfarin
- *Note*: carbamazepine induces hepatic drug-metabolising enzymes; hence a wide range of further interactions exists

Route of administration
- Oral, rectal (for epilepsy, if oral route not possible)

Note
- It is important to start therapy with a low dose in order to minimise adverse effects. The dose is then increased in small increments every 2 weeks until symptoms are controlled.
- It is recommended to monitor blood count, hepatic function and renal function whilst on carbamazepine therapy.
- Carbamazepine can cause folate deficiency. It may cause neural tube defects or hypospadias in the fetus.
- Carbamazepine can induce its own metabolism.
- Therapeutic drug monitoring is recommended.

Related drugs
- Oxcarbazepine

Chlorpromazine

Class: Phenothiazine

Indications
- Psychotic disorders (e.g. schizophrenia, mania)
- Labyrinthine disturbances and vertigo
- Nausea and vomiting
- Chronic hiccups

Mechanism of action
- Exact mechanism is not fully understood.
- In psychotic disorders chlorpromazine is thought to block D_2 receptors in the CNS, especially in the mesocortical and mesolimbic areas.
- The antiemetic effect is due to blockade of dopamine receptors in the chemoreceptor trigger zone in the brain.
- Blockade of muscarinic, histamine 1, serotonin and alpha receptors might contribute to the therapeutic action of chlorpromazine, but blockade of these also causes adverse effects.

Adverse effects
- *Common*: sedation, postural hypotension, raised prolactin levels (leading to subfertility, impotence, menstrual disturbances, galactorrhoea), extrapyramidal adverse effects (acute dystonia, akathisia, Parkinsonism, tardive dyskinesia with long-term use), anticholinergic effects (e.g. dry mouth, blurred vision)
- *Rare*: neuroleptic malignant syndrome (hyperthermia, muscle rigidity, autonomic nervous system dysfunction), agranulocytosis, photosensitive rash, jaundice

Contraindications
- Coma
- Bone marrow suppression
- Phaeochromocytoma
- Pregnancy and breastfeeding

Interactions
- *ACE inhibitors*: these can cause severe postural hypotension if given with chlorpromazine

Route of administration
- Oral, rectal, IM

Note
- Compliance may be a problem in psychotic patients. In this case slow-release preparations of other neuroleptics (e.g. haloperidol decanoate) can be given IM every few weeks.
- Extrapyramidal adverse effects are thought to be due to the blockade of dopamine receptors in the CNS.
- Chlorpromazine can be used in conjunction with an anticholinergic drug (e.g. procyclidine) to prevent short-term extrapyramidal adverse effects. This, however, cannot prevent tardive dyskinesia.

Related drugs
- Fluphenazine, levomepromazine, perphenazine, pevicyazine, pipothiazine, prochlorperazine, thioridazine, trifluoperazine

Diazepam

Class: Benzodiazepine

Indications
- Anxiety
- Status epilepticus
- Febrile convulsions
- Muscle spasm (e.g. spasticity)

Mechanism of action
- Diazepam facilitates opening of chloride channels in the CNS by binding to the GABA/chloride-channel complex. The resulting flow of chloride ions results in hyperpolarisation and therefore neuronal inhibition. It is thought that this action produces the anxiolytic, anticonvulsant and sedative effects.

Adverse effects
- *Common*: daytime drowsiness, confusion in the elderly
- *Rare*: headache, blurred vision, confusion, rash, thrombophlebitis (with IV injection), respiratory depression, apnoea

Contraindications
- Respiratory depression
- Sleep apnoea
- Severe hepatic impairment
- Myasthenia gravis
- Chronic psychosis

Interactions
- *Isoniazid*: this inhibits the metabolism of diazepam
- *Rifampicin*: this increases the metabolism of diazepam
- *Sedatives*: any other sedative may enhance the sedative effect of diazepam

Route of administration
- Oral, rectal (if oral route inappropriate), IM or IV (status epilepticus, acute severe anxiety)

Note
- Diazepam is metabolised by the liver to active metabolites that have very long half-lives (e.g. *N*-desmethyl diazepam has a half-life of up to 200 h). Accumulation of active metabolites can therefore easily occur.
- Flumazenil is a specific benzodiazepine antagonist that can be given in benzodiazepine overdose, but may precipitate a withdrawal syndrome.

Related drugs
- Alprazolam, clobazam, clonazepam, flunitrazepam, flurazepam, nitrazepam

Fluoxetine

Class: Selective serotonin reuptake inhibitor (SSRI)

Indications
- Depression
- Obsessive–compulsive disorder
- Bulimia nervosa

Mechanism of action
- Fluoxetine increases serotonin levels in the CNS by inhibiting its reuptake from the synaptic cleft.

Adverse effects
- *Common*: headache, insomnia, nausea, diarrhoea, anxiety, sexual dysfunction
- *Rare*: anaphylaxis, drowsiness, serotonin syndrome (agitation, confusion, fever, trembling), constipation

Contraindications
- Mania

Interactions
- *Carbamazepine*: fluoxetine increases the plasma concentration of carbamazepine
- *Dopaminergics*: fluoxetine causes hypertension and CNS excitation if given with dopaminergics
- *Lithium*: fluoxetine increases the risk of lithium toxicity
- *Phenytoin*: fluoxetine increases the plasma concentration of phenytoin

Route of administration
- Oral

Note
- SSRIs are preferred to TCAs because they are safer in overdose. They are relatively free of anticholinergic adverse effects such as blurred vision, dry mouth and difficult micturition. They are also less sedating than TCAs and less cardiotoxic.
- After stopping fluoxetine, active substances may persist in the body for weeks. This must be borne in mind when prescribing new drugs that may interact with fluoxetine after having discontinued it.
- Fluoxetine should not be started until 14 days after stopping an MAOI.

Related drugs
- Citalopram, fluvoxamine, paroxetine, sertraline

Haloperidol

Class: Butyrophenone dopamine 2 antagonist

Indications
- Schizophrenia and other psychotic disorders
- Motor tics
- Short-term sedation of acutely violent or otherwise agitated patients (e.g. in dementia)

Mechanism of action
- Haloperidol blocks postsynaptic dopamine 2 receptors in the limbic, striatal and cortical brain regions.
- It also blocks dopamine 1 receptors, but to a much lesser extent.

Adverse effects
- *Common*: extrapyramidal effects with long-term use (e.g. Parkinsonism, acute dystonia, akathisia), drowsiness, postural hypotension
- *Rare*: weight loss, tardive dyskinesia, convulsions, neuroleptic malignant syndrome

Contraindications
- Coma
- Bone marrow depression

Interactions
- *Amiodarone*: haloperidol increases the risk of ventricular dysrhythmias if given with amiodarone
- *Carbamazepine*: this decreases the plasma concentration of haloperidol by accelerating its metabolism
- *Fluoxetine*: this increases the plasma concentration of haloperidol

Route of administration
- Oral, IM

Note
- Haloperidol requires several weeks to exert control over the symptoms of schizophrenia.
- Extrapyramidal adverse effects (e.g. Parkinsonism, akathisia) can be ameliorated by giving muscarinic antagonists (e.g. procyclidine) or by dose reduction.
- In order to avoid first-pass metabolism and improve compliance, haloperidol can be given every 1–4 weeks as a long-acting, deep depot IM injection (given as haloperidol decanoate).
- Haloperidol, as well as any other neuroleptic agent, can cause the potentially fatal neuroleptic malignant syndrome: hyperpyrexia, confusion, increased muscle tone and autonomic dysfunction. There is no effective treatment for this apart from immediate discontinuation of the causative drug.

Related drugs
- Benperidol, droperidol

Hyoscine

Class: Muscarinic antagonist

Indications
- Prophylaxis of motion sickness
- Intestinal or renal colic
- Premedication (in anaesthesia)
- Eye examination (to dilate pupils)

Mechanism of action
- Hyoscine competes with acetylcholine for muscarinic receptors. This results in:
  1 Smooth muscle relaxation in bowel, bladder and ureters
  2 Reduced secretions from bronchial and sweat glands
  3 Pupillary dilatation
  4 Bronchodilatation
  5 Increase in heart rate

Adverse effects
- *Common*: sedation, dry mouth, blurred vision, constipation
- *Rare*: difficulty with micturition, confusion, restlessness

Contraindications
- Prostatic hypertrophy
- Closed-angle glaucoma
- Myasthenia gravis
- Paralytic ileus
- Pyloric stenosis

Interactions
- *Alcohol*: this enhances the sedative effect of hyoscine

Route of administration
- IV, IM, oral, skin patch, eye drops, subcutaneous

Note
- Muscarinic adverse effects of hyoscine can be counteracted by anticholinesterase drugs (e.g. neostigmine).
- Hyoscine effectively relaxes the colon and the pyloric antral area in the stomach. These actions are useful to the radiologist and the endoscopist.

Related drugs
- Atropine (less sedating than hyoscine)

Levodopa

Class: Dopamine precursor

Indications
- Idiopathic Parkinson's disease

Mechanism of action
- Levodopa is an aminoacid precursor of dopamine. It crosses the blood–brain barrier and is then converted to dopamine by the enzyme dopa decarboxylase. This action replaces dopamine, which is deficient in the basal ganglia in Parkinson's disease. Dopamine itself is not used in Parkinson's disease as it cannot cross the blood–brain barrier.

Adverse effects
- *Common*:
  - Systemic adverse effects – nausea, vomiting, abdominal pain, anorexia, postural hypotension, dizziness, discoloration of urine and other body fluids
  - CNS adverse effects – abnormal involuntary movements, 'on–off effect' (rigidity alternating with excessive movements)
- *Rare*: psychiatric symptoms (e.g. confusion, hallucinations, depression), cardiac dysrhythmias

Contraindications
- Closed-angle glaucoma
- Drug-induced Parkinsonism

Interactions
- *Anaesthetics*: concomitant use of levodopa and volatile liquid anaesthetics increases the risk of cardiac dysrhythmias
- *MAOIs*: risk of hypertensive crisis (withdraw MAOIs two weeks before starting levodopa)
- *Neuroleptics*: these reduce the effects of levodopa by blocking dopamine receptors

Route of administration
- Oral

Note
- Only 1–5% of levodopa reaches the brain as it is peripherally converted to dopamine by dopa decarboxylase. Combining levodopa with a decarboxylase inhibitor such as benserazide or carbidopa can prevent this. Thus more dopamine reaches the brain and a reduction in systemic adverse effects is achieved.
- The efficacy of levodopa decreases with long-term use.
- Anticholinergic drugs (e.g. benzhexol) may be helpful in controlling tremor and excess salivation that occur in Parkinson's disease.

Lithium

Class: Mood stabiliser

Indications
- Treatment and prophylaxis of mania
- Bipolar affective disorder
- Resistant recurrent depression

Mechanism of action
- Exact mechanism is not fully understood.
- Lithium is thought to:
  1 reduce glutamatergic activity in the CNS;
  2 act upon signal mechanisms in the CNS (adenylyl cyclase, glycogen synthase kinase-3 beta, cyclic AMP); and
  3 inhibit second messengers in the CNS.
- All these actions are believed to assist in stabilising neuronal activity.

Adverse effects
- *Common*: weight gain, nausea, vomiting, diarrhoea, tremor
- *Rare*: renal tubular damage (nephrogenic diabetes insipidus, interstitial nephritis), hypothyroidism, muscle weakness, drowsiness, blurred vision, rash, memory impairment (in long-term use), cardiac dysrhythmias

Contraindications
- None
- Caution:
  - Renal impairment (lithium is excreted renally)
  - Cardiac disease
  - Pregnancy and breastfeeding
  - Elderly

Interactions
- *Diuretics*: these increase the plasma concentration of lithium by reducing its excretion
- *SSRIs*: these increase the risk of lithium adverse effects

Route of administration
- Oral

Note
- An ECG should be taken prior to starting lithium (risk of cardiac dysrhythmias).
- Thyroid and renal function must be tested prior to and during treatment with lithium because of its potential nephrotoxic and thyrotoxic effects.
- Lithium has a narrow therapeutic window. Plasma concentration must therefore be monitored, as overdose can be fatal.
- Lithium toxicity manifests as drowsiness, confusion, ataxia, seizures and coma. Management of toxicity includes increasing fluid intake and providing supportive treatment. Haemodialysis can be performed in severe cases.
- Sodium competes with lithium for reabsorption in the renal tubules. Hyponatraemia can therefore increase the risk of lithium toxicity.

Phenelzine

Class: Monoamine oxidase inhibitor (MAOI)

Indications
- Depression
- Phobic states

Mechanism of action
- Phenelzine causes non-selective irreversible inhibition of the enzyme monoamine oxidase type A, which is involved in the metabolism of serotonin, norepinephrine and dopamine. This results in increased concentrations of these neurotransmitters in the brain, peripheral neurones, gut wall and platelets.
- Monoamine oxidase in the gut wall normally metabolises tyramine in foodstuffs. If tyramine-containing food is ingested whilst on phenelzine, this can lead to an accumulation of tyramine, which in turn causes a rise in norepinephrine levels. This can trigger a hypertensive crisis.

Adverse effects
- *Common*: dizziness, dry mouth, blurred vision, postural hypotension
- *Rare*: hypertensive crisis, hepatotoxicity, rash, drowsiness, constipation

Contraindications
- Hepatic impairment
- Cerebrovascular disease
- Phaeochromocytoma

Interactions
- *Levodopa and sympathomimetics*: increased risk of a hypertensive crisis (sweating, restlessness, flushing, hyperpyrexia, tremor, convulsions, coma)
- *TCAs*: predisposition to CNS excitation and hypertension
- *Tyramine-containing foods (e.g. pickled herring, cheese, wine, beer, yeast, chocolate)*: risk of a hypertensive crisis

Route of administration
- Oral

Note
- Due to its drug and food interactions (especially with tyramine-rich foods) phenelzine is usually a 3rd line drug for the treatment of depression after TCAs and SSRIs.
- MAOIs should not be started until at least 2 weeks after a previous MAOI, TCA or SSRI has been stopped (5 weeks for fluoxetine, due to longer half-life).
- Other antidepressants should not be started for 2 weeks after treatment with an MAOI has been stopped.
- Patients should carry a warning card, detailing which foods should be avoided (see above under *Interactions*).
- Phenelzine is metabolised by acetylation. Slow acetylators (about half the population of Europe and the USA) are more likely to develop adverse effects.

Related drugs
- Isocarboxazid, tranylcypromine

Phenytoin

Class: Anticonvulsant

Indications
- All types of epilepsy except absence seizures
- Trigeminal neuralgia

Mechanism of action
- Phenytoin alters transmembrane movement of Na^+ and K^+ by blocking voltage-gated Na^+ channels. This action stabilises neuronal thresholds against hyperexcitability.
- Phenytoin acts primarily in the motor cortex of the brain. It is thought to prevent the spread of epileptic discharges, not the initiation.

Adverse effects
- *Common*: dizziness, insomnia, nausea, vomiting, coarsening of facial features, hirsutism, acne
- *Rare*: gum hypertrophy, Stevens–Johnson syndrome, drug-induced SLE, peripheral neuropathy, Dupuytren's contracture, hepatitis, cardiac dysrhythmias, folic acid or vitamin D deficiency

Contraindications
- None
- Caution:
  - Pregnancy and breastfeeding

Interactions
- *Amiodarone, cimetidine, diltiazem*: these drugs increase the plasma concentration of phenytoin
- *Oral contraceptive pill*: phenytoin decreases the effect of the oral contraceptive pill by increasing its metabolism
- *Warfarin*: phenytoin increases the metabolism of warfarin
- *Note*: Phenytoin induces hepatic drug-metabolising enzymes; hence a wide range of further interactions exists

Route of administration
- Oral (epilepsy, trigeminal neuralgia), IV (epilepsy)

Note
- Phenytoin has a narrow therapeutic window and a non-linear relationship between dose and plasma concentration (zero-order kinetics). It therefore requires therapeutic drug monitoring.
- Patients should be advised how to recognise signs of phenytoin toxicity (mostly CNS effects: tremor, nystagmus, ataxia, dysarthria and convulsions).
- Due to cosmetic adverse effects, phenytoin may be undesirable for use in adolescents.
- Phenytoin is teratogenic and is associated with congenital heart disease and cleft palate/lip. Antenatal screening is recommended.
- If phenytoin is given IV, cardiac monitoring is essential (risk of dysrhythmias).

Related drugs
- Fosphenytoin (a prodrug of phenytoin)

Risperidone

Class: Benzisoxazole derivative ('atypical' neuroleptic)

Indications
- Psychosis (acute or chronic)

Mechanism of action
- Exact mechanism is not fully understood.
- Risperidone is believed to achieve its effect by blocking D_2 and 5-HT_2 receptors in the brain. It may also block other receptors, thus contributing to some of the adverse effects.

Adverse effects
- *Common*: headache, anxiety, insomnia, postural hypotension, extrapyramidal symptoms (restlessness, tremor, muscle stiffness)
- *Rare*: constipation, postural hypotension, tardive dyskinesia, neuroleptic malignant syndrome, blurred vision, cardiac dysrhythmias, hyperprolactinaemia

Contraindications
- Breastfeeding

Interactions
- *Carbamazepine*: increased metabolism of risperidone
- *Fluoxetine*: raised plasma concentration of risperidone

Route of administration
- Oral

Note
- Risperidone is especially useful for controlling 'negative' as well as 'positive' symptoms in psychosis.
- Before starting treatment with risperidone, an ECG should be taken. When established on treatment, blood pressure should be checked regularly.
- Full benefits of risperidone begin to show after 1–2 weeks of treatment.

Related drugs
- Other 'atypical' neuroleptics: clozapine, olanzapine, quetiapine, zotepine

Sodium valproate

Class: Anticonvulsant

Indications
- All types of epilepsy

Mechanism of action
- Sodium valproate increases GABA content of the brain by inhibiting the enzyme GABA transaminase and preventing GABA reuptake.
- Sodium valproate also reduces concentrations of aspartate, an excitatory neurotransmitter.
- In addition, it blocks voltage-gated sodium channels.

Adverse effects
- *Common*: nausea, vomiting, weight gain
- *Rare*: hepatic failure, pancreatitis, blood dyscrasias (pancytopenia, thrombocytopenia, leucopenia), sedation, transient hair loss

Contraindications
- Hepatic dysfunction (sodium valproate is metabolised and excreted by the liver)
- Porphyria

Interactions
- *Anticonvulsants*: two or more anticonvulsants given together may lead to enhanced effects, increased sedation or reduced plasma concentrations of either drug
- *Neuroleptics*: neuroleptics decrease the anticonvulsant effect of sodium valproate
- *Tricyclic antidepressants*: these decrease the anticonvulsant effect of sodium valproate

Route of administration
- Oral, IV

Note
- Liver function tests should be carried out regularly.
- Sodium valproate is especially useful in children with atonic epilepsy or absence seizures as it has little sedative effect.
- Sodium valproate has fewer adverse effects than most other anticonvulsants.
- Patients should be given an information leaflet describing how to recognise haematological and hepatic adverse effects of sodium valproate.
- Sodium valproate is teratogenic and is associated with congenital abnormalities, including spina bifida. Counselling and antenatal screening are recommended, as well as regular folate for pregnant women on sodium valproate.

Sumatriptan

Class: Serotonin (5-HT$_1$) agonist

Indications
- Acute migraine
- Cluster headache (subcutaneous use only)

Mechanism of action
- Sumatriptan selectively stimulates the inhibitory serotonin (5-HT$_1$) receptors in the raphe nucleus of the brain. It thereby maintains vasoconstrictor tone, which mainly occurs in the carotid arterial circulation. This action is believed to reduce the severity of acute migraine attacks.

Adverse effects
- *Common*: pain at the injection site, flushing, lethargy, tingling
- *Rare*: chest pain, dizziness

Contraindications
- Ischaemic heart disease (sumatriptan produces a small degree of vasoconstriction in coronary vessels)
- Severe hypertension

Interactions
- *Ergotamine*: concomitant use of ergotamine and sumatriptan increases the risk of vasospasm
- *Lithium*: concomitant use of lithium and sumatriptan increases the risk of CNS toxicity
- *MAOIs*: concomitant use of MAOIs and sumatriptan increases the risk of CNS toxicity
- *SSRIs*: concomitant use of SSRIs and sumatriptan increases the risk of CNS toxicity

Route of administration
- Oral, intranasal spray, subcutaneous

Note
- In acute migraine simple analgesics such as paracetamol should be tried first. If these are ineffective, sumatriptan can be used.
- Sumatriptan should be given as soon as possible after the onset of a migraine attack.
- It is more effective if given subcutaneously.
- Sumatriptan is recommended as monotherapy (concomitant use with other antimigraine drugs should be avoided).

Related drugs
- Naratriptan, rizatriptan, zolmitriptan

Temazepam

Class: Benzodiazepine

Indications
- Insomnia
- Premedication before surgery

Mechanism of action
- Temazepam binds to GABA receptors in the CNS and thereby facilitates GABA-inhibitory neurotransmission by opening chloride channels. This action is thought to produce the sedative and anxiolytic effects.

Adverse effects
- *Common*: dependence (with prolonged use)
- *Rare*: seizures, drowsiness, ataxia, anxiety, nightmares, rash, agitation, headache

Contraindications
- Respiratory depression (may be worsened by temazepam)
- Severe hepatic impairment
- Myasthenia gravis
- Sleep apnoea syndrome

Interactions
- *Alcohol*: this enhances the sedative effect of temazepam
- *Cimetidine*: this inhibits the metabolism of temazepam

Route of administration
- Oral

Note
- Sedative and anxiolytic effects of temazepam last for about 90 min.
- Temazepam should be used short term only to avoid psychological and physical dependence.
- Flumazenil can be used as antidote to temazepam overdose or to reverse its effects.

Related drugs
- Loprazolam, lorazepam, lormetazepam, midazolam, oxazepam

Zopiclone

Class: Cyclopyrrolone hypnotic

Indications
- Insomnia

Mechanism of action
- Zopiclone acts in a similar way to benzodiazepines but causes less sedation, less dependence and less muscle relaxation.
- It binds to the benzodiazepine receptor complex in the CNS, which facilitates the actions of GABA, an inhibitory neurotransmitter.

Adverse effects
- *Common*: bitter taste in mouth, GI effects (anorexia, abdominal pain, constipation)
- *Rare*: mood changes, dependence (with long-term use), palpitations, agitation, trembling

Contraindications
- Myasthenia gravis
- Respiratory failure
- Severe sleep apnoea
- Severe hepatic impairment
- Pregnancy and breastfeeding

Interactions
- *Erythromycin*: this inhibits the metabolism of zopiclone

Route of administration
- Oral

Note
- Non-drug therapy should be tried prior to starting zopiclone.
- Zopiclone increases the duration of sleep and reduces the number of nocturnal awakenings.
- Overdose manifests as confusion, ataxia and drowsiness. This should be managed with gastric lavage, IV fluids and observation.
- Continuous treatment with zopiclone should not exceed 2–4 weeks. Continued use may result in dependence.
- Zopiclone causes less 'morning-after' drowsiness than long-acting benzodiazepines.

Related drugs
- Zaleplon, zolpidem

MUSCULOSKELETAL SYSTEM

Management guidelines (pp. 89–90)
Gout
Osteoarthritis
Osteoporosis
Rheumatoid arthritis

Drug classes (p. 91)
Corticosteroids

Individual drugs (pp. 92 100)
Alendronic acid; Allopurinol; Azathioprine; Celecoxib;
Ciclosporin; Cyclophosphamide; Methotrexate; Penicillamine;
Prednisolone

GOUT
Acute gout
• In an acute attack give an NSAID (e.g. indomethacin) but *not*
aspirin, as it inhibits uric acid excretion
• If NSAIDs are contraindicated, give colchicine or IM depot
injection of corticosteroids

Prevention of gout
• Reduce excessive alcohol intake and purine-rich foods (oily
fish, liver, kidney)
• Encourage weight loss if appropriate
• Consider allopurinol to decrease uric acid synthesis, or a
uricosuric drug (i.e. probenecid, sulfinpyrazone) to increase
urinary uric acid excretion

OSTEOARTHRITIS
• Recommend regular physical exercise to maintain muscle
bulk and joint mobility
• Reduce weight if appropriate
• Supply walking aid if necessary
• Paracetamol and NSAIDs for pain control
• Intra-articular steroid injections are useful for inflammatory
exacerbations
• Consider joint replacement if pain and loss of joint function
do not respond to analgesics and exercise

OSTEOPOROSIS
Prevention
• Advise lifestyle measures such as regular exercise, cessation of
smoking, avoiding excess alcohol, and avoiding immobility

- Maintain adequate calcium and vitamin D intake. Give supplements if necessary.
- In the frail elderly, consider hip protector pants to prevent fractures from falls

Treatment
- Confirm osteoporosis with bone densitometry
- Advise lifestyle changes (as above)
- Give a bisphosphonate (e.g. alendronic acid) or raloxifene (selective oestrogen receptor modulator) with calcium and vitamin D supplementation
- Calcitonin may be used in some cases

RHEUMATOID ARTHRITIS
- Multidisciplinary team approach is important (education, physiotherapy, joint protection, walking aids, orthotics, social services, GP and specialist)
- Recommend regular physical exercise to maintain muscle bulk and joint mobility

Medical treatment
- 1st line therapy:
  - Disease-modifying antirheumatic drugs (methotrexate and sometimes sulfasalazine) slow disease progression and alter inflammatory markers but require monitoring
  - Paracetamol and NSAIDs for symptomatic relief (e.g. ibuprofen, celecoxib)
- 2nd line therapy: alternative DMARDs (i.e. penicillamine, gold, hydroxychloroquine, azathioprine, ciclosporin)
- Antitumour necrosis factor antibodies (i.e. infliximab, etanercept) can be used for active disease not responding to two or more conventional DMARDs
- Corticosteroids can be given for an anti-inflammatory effect:
  - Orally
  - Parenterally – IM long-acting depot injection or large bolus given IV
  - Locally – injection into an inflamed joint

Surgical treatment
- Surgery is an option for some patients (e.g. carpal tunnel decompression, synovectomy, tendon repair, arthrodesis, arthroplasty)

CORTICOSTEROIDS
Types of corticosteroids
1 Glucocorticoids: beclomethasone, cortisone, dexamethasone, hydrocortisone, methylprednisolone, prednisolone, triamcinolone
2 Mineralocorticoids (these have a much weaker effect than glucocorticoids): fludrocortisone

Indications
1 Glucocorticoids are mainly used for:
  • Suppression of inflammation
  • Suppression of the immune system
  • Replacement therapy
  • Part of chemotherapy (in Hodgkin's lymphoma and acute leukaemia)
  • Reduction of oedema (e.g. in brain tumours)
2 Mineralocorticoids are mainly used in replacement therapy

Adverse effects
• Glucocorticoid effects: Cushingoid appearance, osteoporosis, growth suppression, diabetes mellitus, peptic ulcer, cataract, glaucoma, susceptibility to infection, impaired wound healing, easy bruising
• Mineralocorticoid effects: hypokalaemia and hypertension (secondary to sodium and water retention)
• *Note*: Topical use of corticosteroids limits systemic adverse effects

Alendronic acid

Class: Bisphosphonate

Indications
- Prevention and treatment of osteoporosis

Mechanism of action
- Alendronic acid inhibits osteoclast activity and hence reduces bone turnover. It improves bone mineralisation and increases bone mass.
- Alendronic acid is thought to achieve its effects through inhibition of a rate-limiting step in cholesterol synthesis, which is essential for the normal function of osteoclasts.

Adverse effects
- *Common*: abdominal discomfort, flatulence, headache
- *Rare*: oesophagitis, oesophageal strictures, peptic ulceration, hypocalcaemia

Contraindications
- Oesophageal abnormalities (e.g. achalasia, stricture)
- Pregnancy and breastfeeding
- Hypocalcaemia

Interactions
- *Aminoglycosides*: these increase the risk of hypocalcaemia

Route of administration
- Oral

Note
- Other bisphosphonates (e.g. disodium pamidronate) can be used for the treatment of Paget's disease of bone and hypercalcaemia of malignancy.
- Alendronic acid has been shown to prevent fractures due to postmenopausal and corticosteroid-induced osteoporosis.

Related drugs
- Disodium etidronate, disodium pamidronate, ibandronic acid, risedronate sodium, sodium clodronate, tiludronic acid, zoledronic acid

Allopurinol

Class: Anti-gout agent

Indications
- Prophylaxis of gout
- Prophylaxis of uric acid and calcium oxalate renal stones
- Prophylaxis of hyperuricaemia secondary to chemotherapy

Mechanism of action
- Allopurinol decreases uric acid production by inhibiting the enzyme xanthine oxidase, which converts xanthine to uric acid. The excess xanthine is easily excreted as it is more soluble.

Adverse effects
- *Rare*. hypersensitivity, rash, headache, metallic taste in the mouth, blood disorders, Stevens–Johnson syndrome

Contraindications
- Acute gout attack
- Caution:
  - Renal impairment (allopurinol is renally excreted)

Interactions
- *Ampicillin*: increased risk of a rash
- *Azathioprine, mercaptopurine*: the effects of these drugs are enhanced by allopurinol
- *Warfarin*: allopurinol may enhance the effect of warfarin

Route of administration
- Oral

Note
- The risk of a gout attack is increased in the first few weeks of treatment with allopurinol. This can be avoided by taking allopurinol with an NSAID (not aspirin) or colchicine.
- High fluid intake during allopurinol therapy is recommended (approximately 2 L/day).

Azathioprine

Class: Immunosuppressive agent

Indications
- Autoimmune diseases (e.g. rheumatoid arthritis, SLE)
- Prevention of transplant rejection
- Used as a steroid-sparing drug (to allow lower doses of corticosteroids in severe inflammatory conditions)

Mechanism of action
- Azathioprine is metabolised to 6-mercaptopurine in the liver. This metabolite is taken up into cells, where it inhibits DNA synthesis. Azathioprine thus has a cytotoxic effect on dividing cells.

Adverse effects
- *Common*: nausea, vomiting, bone marrow suppression
- *Rare*: alopecia, arthralgia, liver impairment, pancreatitis, renal impairment

Contraindications
- Hypersensitivity

Interactions
- *Allopurinol*: this inhibits the metabolism of azathioprine, thus increasing the risk of adverse effects
- *Antibacterials*: risk of toxicity of azathioprine is enhanced with rifampicin, co-trimoxazole and trimethoprim
- *Warfarin*: effect of warfarin possibly reduced

Route of administration
- Oral, IV (very irritant and only rarely used)

Note
- Azathioprine is potentially highly toxic. Close monitoring is required, whereby FBC is checked regularly to detect bone marrow suppression.
- Bone marrow suppression may manifest as bleeding, bruising, fatigue or repeated infections.
- The standard dose of azathioprine should be reduced in the elderly and patients with renal or hepatic impairment.

Celecoxib

Class: Non-steroidal anti-inflammatory drug (NSAID); COX-2 inhibitor

Indications
- Inflammation and pain in rheumatoid and osteoarthritis

Mechanism of action
- Celecoxib inhibits conversion of arachidonic acid into prostaglandin E_2 through selective inhibition of COX-2. This leads to:
  1 a decrease in vascular permeability and vasodilatation (anti-inflammatory effect);
  2 a decrease in sensitisation of pain afferents (analgesic effect); and
  3 a decrease in the effect of prostaglandins on the hypothalamus (antipyretic effect).
- COX-1 inhibition is associated with GI adverse effects. Since celecoxib is a specific COX-2 inhibitor, such adverse effects are rare (especially when compared to other NSAIDs).

Adverse effects
- *Common*: abdominal discomfort, insomnia, sinusitis
- *Rare*: palpitations, GI bleeding, stomatitis, muscle cramps

Contraindications
- Active peptic ulceration
- Inflammatory bowel disease

Interactions
- *Fluconazole*: plasma concentration of celecoxib is increased by fluconazole

Route of administration
- Oral

Note
- COX-2 inhibitors have a lower risk of upper GI bleeding than non-selective NSAIDs. Other adverse effects are similar to those of non-selective NSAIDs.
- Celecoxib may be used with caution in patients with a past history of peptic ulcers or GI bleeding.
- COX-2 inhibitors should be used in preference to non-selective NSAIDs in patients at increased risk of GI bleeding.
- Unlike aspirin, celecoxib has no anti-platelet properties.
- Rofecoxib has been withdrawn as it has been associated with an increased incidence of ischaemic events (e.g. MI, stroke).

Related drugs
- Other COX-2 inhibitors: etodolac, etoricoxib, meloxicam, valdecoxib

Ciclosporin

Class: Immunosuppressive agent

Indications
- Severe rheumatoid arthritis
- Prevention of transplant rejection
- Prophylaxis and treatment of graft-versus-host disease
- Nephrotic syndrome
- Severe eczema and psoriasis (when conventional therapy has failed)

Mechanism of action
- Ciclosporin is an immunosuppressive agent directed mainly against T lymphocytes. It prevents their activation and reduces the release of cytokines, in particular interleukin-2. This action suppresses cell-mediated immunity and to a lesser extent antibody-mediated immunity.

Adverse effects
- *Common*: nephrotoxicity, hypertension
- *Rare*: hirsutism, gum hypertrophy, convulsions, muscle weakness, hepatic impairment

Contraindications
- Renal disease
- Liver disease
- Uncontrolled hypertension
- Malignancy

Interactions
- *Aminoglycosides, erythromycin, trimethoprim*: these drugs increase plasma ciclosporin levels, thus increasing the risk of nephrotoxicity
- *Carbamazepine, phenytoin, rifampicin*: these drugs reduce the plasma concentration of ciclosporin
- *Diltiazem, verapamil*: these drugs increase the plasma concentration of ciclosporin, thus increasing the risk of nephrotoxicity
- *NSAIDs*: concomitant use of NSAIDs and cyclosporin increases the risk of nephrotoxicity

Route of administration
- Oral, IV

Note
- Unlike other immunosuppressive agents, ciclosporin does not cause bone marrow suppression.
- Therapeutic drug monitoring is required.
- Some evidence suggests that patients taking ciclosporin are at an increased risk of secondary lymphomas caused by EBV infection. This is believed to be due to impaired immunity.

Cyclophosphamide

Class: Alkylating agent (immunosuppressive agent)

Indications
- Malignant tumours (lymphomas, chronic lymphocytic leukaemia and solid tumours)
- Vasculitis
- Autoimmune disease (e.g. SLE)

Mechanism of action
- Cyclophosphamide is inactive until it undergoes hepatic metabolism.
- It damages the DNA in cells by forming cross-links between strands and by causing base substitution. Consequently, the DNA cannot replicate and this prevents cell division.

Adverse effects
- *Common*: bone marrow suppression, alopecia, and in high dose: nausea, vomiting, anorexia
- *Rare*: haemorrhagic cystitis, infertility in men (with long-term use)

Contraindications
- Porphyria

Interactions
- *Suxamethonium*: the effects of suxamethonium are enhanced by cyclophosphamide

Route of administration
- Oral, IV

Note
- Whilst on cyclophosphamide, it is recommended to be taking mesna and to maintain a high fluid intake in order to prevent haemorrhagic cystitis. Mesna neutralises acrolein, the toxic metabolite of cyclophosphamide, which damages the bladder. Mesna should be continued for about 24–48 h after stopping cyclophosphamide.
- As cyclophosphamide acts on the testis, long-term treatment may lead to infertility by decreasing the sperm count. This may be irreversible and a discussion regarding sperm storage should therefore be undertaken with the patient before therapy.
- Long-term use may increase the risk of developing acute myeloid leukaemia.

Methotrexate

Class: Immunosuppressive agent

Indications
- Part of various cancer chemotherapy regimens (e.g. acute lymphoblastic leukaemia, non-Hodgkin's lymphoma, choriocarcinoma)
- Rheumatoid arthritis
- Psoriasis (when conventional therapy has failed)

Mechanism of action
- Methotrexate is a competitive antagonist of the enzyme dihydrofolate reductase, which catalyses the production of tetrahydrofolic acid from dihydrofolate. This antagonism results in decreased production of tetrahydrofolic acid, which is an essential component for synthesis of nucleic acids (purines and thymidylic acid). Methotrexate therefore inhibits DNA, RNA and protein synthesis, leading to cell death.
- Methotrexate further suppresses epidermal activity in the skin, hence its use in psoriasis.

Adverse effects
- *Common*: bone marrow suppression, mucositis (e.g. stomatitis, gingivitis), anorexia, nausea, vomiting, diarrhoea, hepatotoxicity (with prolonged treatment)
- *Rare*: pneumonitis, pulmonary fibrosis

Contraindications
- Renal impairment (methotrexate is renally excreted)
- Hepatic impairment
- Pregnancy and breastfeeding
- Immunodeficiency syndromes

Interactions
- *Acitretin*: this increases the plasma concentration of methotrexate, thus increasing the risk of hepatotoxicity
- *Ciclosporin*: this increases methotrexate toxicity
- *NSAIDs*: these increase the risk of methotrexate toxicity by reducing its excretion
- *Probenecid*: this increases the risk of methotrexate toxicity by reducing its excretion

Route of administration
- Oral, IM, IV, intrathecal

Note
- Folinic acid is used to prevent and reverse the toxic effects of methotrexate ('folinic acid rescue').
- Methotrexate has teratogenic effects. Contraceptive precautions are therefore necessary during and until 3 months after stopping treatment with methotrexate.
- Treatment with methotrexate can cause folate deficiency leading to megaloblastic anaemia.

Penicillamine

Class: Disease-modifying antirheumatic drug (DMARD)

Indications
- Wilson's disease
- Copper poisoning
- Lead poisoning
- Cystinuria
- Active rheumatoid arthritis

Mechanism of action
- Exact mechanism in rheumatoid arthritis is not fully understood. Penicillamine has immune-modulatory effects by reducing the number of lymphocytes.
- Penicillamine chelates metal ions via its sulphadryl group (hence useful in Wilson's disease and copper/lead poisoning).
- Penicillamine is thought to form a soluble disulphide complex with cystine (hence useful in cystinuria).

Adverse effects
- *Common*: rash, proteinuria, anorexia, nausea, vomiting
- *Rare*: bone marrow suppression, drug-induced lupus, pemphigus, fever, mouth ulceration, myasthenia gravis, loss of taste

Contraindications
- Hypersensitivity to penicillin (penicillamine is a degradation product of penicillin)
- SLE

Interactions
- *Iron*: oral iron reduces the absorption of penicillamine

Route of administration
- Oral

Note
- In rheumatoid arthritis, penicillamine is only used if other drugs have failed.
- Clinical improvement in rheumatoid arthritis can be expected after 6–12 weeks of treatment. Penicillamine should be stopped if no improvement is evident within 1 year. It is now rarely used in rheumatoid arthritis.
- Regular blood and urine tests should be performed to detect any bone marrow suppression or proteinuria.
- Penicillamine should be taken before meals to reduce GI adverse effects.
- Penicillamine should only be prescribed in hospitals by doctors who have experience with this drug.

Prednisolone

Class: Glucocorticoid

Indications
- Anti-inflammatory therapy (e.g. inflammatory bowel disease, asthma, eczema)
- Immunosuppressive therapy (e.g. prevention of transplant rejection, acute leukaemia)
- Glucocorticoid replacement therapy (e.g. Addison's disease)

Mechanism of action
- Prednisolone inhibits phospholipase A_2 activity, which is responsible for the production of free arachidonic acid. Arachidonic acid is the precursor for prostaglandin and leukotriene synthesis. Inhibition of this process therefore achieves an anti-inflammatory effect.
- Prednisolone decreases B and T lymphocyte response to antigens, thus achieving an immunosuppressive effect.

Adverse effects
- *Common*: bruising, hirsutism, moon-face, hypertension, weight gain/oedema, impaired glucose tolerance, acne, cataract, glaucoma, osteoporosis, candida infection
- *Rare*: mood changes (e.g. depression), peptic ulcers, muscle weakness, reactivation of tuberculosis, pancreatitis

Contraindications
- Systemic infection

Interactions
- *Ciclosporin*: increased plasma concentration of prednisolone
- *Phenytoin, carbamazepine*: these reduce the effects of prednisolone

Route of administration
- Oral, IM, IV, topical, rectal

Note
- Patients on prednisolone should be given a steroid card.
- Prolonged treatment with prednisolone leads to adrenal atrophy. Abrupt withdrawal may therefore precipitate acute adrenal insufficiency (Addisonian crisis). Patients who have been on prednisolone for longer than 3 weeks should have it withdrawn gradually.
- Glucocorticoids are normally secreted in increased amounts during physiological stress. As prolonged therapy with prednisolone leads to a diminished adrenocortical response, any significant injury (e.g. trauma, surgery) requires temporary compensatory increase in prednisolone dose.
- Prednisolone increases gluconeogenesis, redistributes fat to the face, neck and trunk, and causes protein breakdown in tissues such as skin, muscle and bone.

Related drugs
- Betamethasone, cortisone, dexamethasone, hydrocortisone, methylprednisolone, triamcinolone

ENDOCRINE SYSTEM

Management guidelines (pp. 101–102)
Diabetes mellitus
Complications of diabetes mellitus
Hyperthyroidism
Hypothyroidism

Individual drugs (pp. 103–110)
Calcitonin; Carbimazole; Desmopressin; Gliclazide; Insulin;
Levothyroxine sodium; Metformin; Tamoxifen

DIABETES MELLITUS
Regular exercise and education is important in both types of
diabetes. Address other risk factors such as lipids, BP control,
smoking cessation and alcohol intake if appropriate.

Diabetes mellitus type 1
• Insulin is always required (amount is tailored to the
individual)
• Regular monitoring of blood glucose is required
• Patient compliance and self-management is essential to
maintain optimal glucose levels and thus minimise the risk
of long-term complications (i.e. retinopathy, peripheral
neuropathy, nephropathy)

Diabetes mellitus type 2
• Recommend diet therapy (reduce fat intake, increase intake
of complex carbohydrates such as pasta and potatoes) and
physical exercise
• Oral hypoglycaemics are used when dietary measures have
failed after a 3-month trial
• Sulphonylureas, metformin, acarbose and thiazolidinediones
can be used alone or in combination
• Metformin is the treatment of choice in patients not
responding to diet (unless $BMI < 20 \, kg/m^2$, in which case a
sulphonylurea is the first choice)
• Give insulin if HbA1c remains unacceptably high. Insulin can
be added to oral hypoglycaemics or can substitute them.

COMPLICATIONS OF DIABETES MELLITUS
Hypoglycaemia
• In type 1 diabetes this is usually due to a late meal or
inadequate carbohydrate intake; in type 2 diabetes
hypoglycaemia is most commonly caused by inappropriate
dosing of hypoglycaemic drugs

- If possible, give oral glucose in readily available form (e.g. dextrose tablets)
- If oral glucose not possible or no improvement after giving oral glucose, give 50–100 ml of 50% dextrose IV (if no IV access, give IM glucagon)
- Dextrose is irritant to veins. After giving IV dextrose, flush with 50 ml of N-saline.

Ketoacidosis
- Give IV fluids
- Give insulin by IV infusion (sliding scale) until glucose levels are within normal range and arterial pH has normalised
- Change to subcutaneous insulin when the patient starts eating
- Monitor plasma potassium (administer potassium when it reaches the normal range in order to prevent insulin-induced hypokalaemia)
- Insert nasogastric tube in comatose, vomiting and nauseated patients to prevent aspiration pneumonia
- Investigate the cause of ketoacidosis

Hyperglycaemic hyperosmotic non-ketotic coma
- Give IV fluids (use 0.45% saline if plasma $Na^+ > 150$ mmol/L)
- Give heparin until patient is mobile (to prevent deep venous thrombosis)
- Give insulin until glucose levels are within the normal range
- Monitor plasma potassium (administer potassium if levels fall)
- Investigate the cause

HYPERTHYROIDISM
- Control symptoms of hyperthyroidism with a beta blocker (e.g. propranolol)
- Give an antithyroid agent (e.g. carbimazole)
- If hyperthyroidism persists, oral radioactive iodine can be given
- Consider thyroidectomy in certain situations (e.g. cosmetic reasons, young women planning pregnancy)
- Patients often become hypothyroid after medical or surgical treatment of hyperthyroidism. These patients then need to start thyroxine replacement therapy.
- **Thyrotoxic crisis**: give IV fluids, IV propranolol, IV hydrocortisone, oral iodine and oral carbimazole; also supportive measures such as tepid sponging

HYPOTHYROIDISM
- Thyroxine replacement for life
- Monitor thyroid function at regular intervals to ensure TSH is within the normal range

Calcitonin

Class: Hormone

Indications
- Paget's disease of bone
- Hypercalcaemia
- Bone pain in malignancy
- Treatment of osteoporosis (menopausal and steroid-induced)

Mechanism of action
- Calcitonin lowers serum calcium by two main mechanisms:
  - it decreases bone resorption by inhibiting the activity of osteoclasts and by reducing their number; and
  - it increases renal calcium and phosphate excretion by inhibiting their reabsorption in the tubules.

Adverse effects
- *Common*: nausea, vomiting, flushing
- *Rare*: tingling in the hand, inflammation at the injection site, unpleasant taste in the mouth

Contraindications
- Breastfeeding

Interactions
- None

Route of administration
- IV, IM, subcutaneous, intranasally

Note
- Two types of calcitonin preparations are available: salmon (natural) and salcatonin (synthetic). Both are immunogenic (antibodies can be made against them), but salcatonin is less so and is thus more suitable in long-term therapy.
- Calcium supplements should be given in conjunction with calcitonin.
- If HRT is not tolerated or is inappropriate, a combination of calcitonin, bisphosphonate and calcium supplements can be used to treat osteoporosis.
- In Paget's disease of bone, calcitonin decreases pain and may prevent neurological complications.

Carbimazole

Class: Antithyroid drug

Indications
- Hyperthyroidism

Mechanism of action
- Carbimazole decreases the production of thyroid hormones T3 (tri-iodothyronine) and T4 (thyroxine) in the thyroid gland.
- Carbimazole has several actions. The main action is blocking thyroid iodine trapping and inhibiting the enzyme thyroid peroxidase, which is necessary for thyroid hormone synthesis.
- Carbimazole also has a local immunosuppressive effect on the thyroid gland.

Adverse effects
- *Common*: GI disturbance, headache, rash, pruritus
- *Rare*: Bone marrow suppression (agranulocytosis, pancytopenia), jaundice, alopecia, arthralgia

Contraindications
- None
- Caution:
  - Breastfeeding
  - Pregnancy (low doses should be used, as carbimazole in high dose crosses the placenta and can cause neonatal hypothyroidism or goitre)
  - Hepatic impairment

Interactions
- None

Route of administration
- Oral

Note
- Treatment of Graves' disease should continue for at least 1 year. Recurrence of hyperthyroidism occurs in more than half of the patients, but can be treated with another course of carbimazole.
- All patients must be advised to seek medical help if they develop features of bone marrow suppression (e.g. sore throat, mouth ulcers, bleeding). If a low neutrophil count is confirmed, treatment must be discontinued.
- Regular monitoring of thyroid function is essential. A TSH in the normal range reflects optimal dosing of carbimazole.
- Carbimazole can be replaced with propylthiouracil if adverse effects such as rash and itching cannot be tolerated.

Related drugs
- Propylthiouracil

Desmopressin

Class: Synthetic antidiuretic hormone (ADH) analogue

Indications
- Treatment and diagnosis of pituitary diabetes insipidus
- Primary nocturnal enuresis
- Haemophilia A
- Postoperative polyuria/polydipsia
- Post lumbar puncture headache

Mechanism of action
- Desmopressin mimics the action of ADH.
- It selectively activates V_2 receptors in renal tubular cells. This causes increased reabsorption of water and decreased excretion of sodium and water, thus controlling polyuria and polydipsia.
- In haemophilia, desmopressin increases the plasma concentration of factor VIII.

Adverse effects
- *Common*: dilutional hyponatraemia, fluid retention
- *Rare*: convulsions, abdominal pain, headache; epistaxis and nasal congestion with nasal spray

Contraindications
- None
- Caution:
  - Renal impairment
  - Heart failure
  - Hypertension

Interactions
- *Indometacin*: this potentiates the effects of desmopressin

Route of administration
- Oral, intranasal, IM, IV, subcutaneous

Note
- Desmopressin is used in the water deprivation test to differentiate between pituitary and nephrogenic diabetes insipidus.
- Doses of desmopressin should be adjusted to allow some diuresis in a 24 h period. If dosing is excessive, there is a risk of hyponatraemia-induced convulsions.
- Vasopressin and terlipressin are used in the treatment of variceal bleeding (GI bleed) until definitive treatment is started. Desmopressin cannot be used since it has no vasoconstrictor effect.

Related drugs
- Terlipressin, vasopressin (ADH)

Gliclazide

Class: Sulphonylurea

Indications
- Type 2 diabetes mellitus

Mechanism of action
- Gliclazide stimulates insulin secretion by binding to sulphonylurea receptors and blocking ATP-dependent potassium channels in pancreatic β cells. This causes depolarisation and insulin release.
- Gliclazide also inhibits gluconeogenesis.
- Gliclazide can only be used in the presence of some pancreatic β-cell activity as it requires the presence of endogenous insulin.

Adverse effects
- *Common*: hypoglycaemia, weight gain
- *Rare*: GI disturbance, bone marrow suppression, rash, hepatitis

Contraindications
- Ketoacidosis
- Pregnancy
- Breastfeeding
- Caution:
  - The elderly and patients with hepatic or renal impairment are very susceptible to hypoglycaemia

Interactions
- *Chloramphenicol*: this enhances the hypoglycaemic effect of gliclazide
- *Corticosteroids*: these antagonise the hypoglycaemic effect of gliclazide
- *Fluconazole, miconazole*: these increase the plasma concentration of gliclazide
- *Loop diuretics, thiazides*: these antagonise the hypoglycaemic effect

Route of administration
- Oral

Note
- Gliclazide is used in non-obese patients with type 2 diabetes mellitus not responding to diet alone.
- Gliclazide is often combined with metformin in those who cannot achieve adequate glycaemic control with either of these two drugs alone. Gliclazide can also be combined with acarbose or insulin.
- As sulphonylureas do not provide adequate glycaemic control during surgery, pregnancy and illness (e.g. infection, MI, trauma), they are usually temporarily substituted with insulin for these events.

Related drugs
- Glibenclamide, glimepiride, glipizide, gliquidone, tolbutamide

Insulin

Class: Peptide hormone

Indications
- Diabetes mellitus types 1 and 2
- Ketoacidosis
- Hyperglycaemic hyperosmotic non-ketotic coma
- Emergency treatment of hyperkalaemia (IV glucose must be co-administered)

Mechanism of action
- Insulin lowers plasma glucose concentration by:
  1 stimulating glucose transport into fat and muscle cells;
  2 stimulating glycogen synthesis; and
  3 inhibiting gluconeogenesis, lipolysis and protein breakdown.

Adverse effects
- *Common*: hypoglycaemia, weight gain
- *Rare*: fat hypertrophy or atrophy at the injection site (sites should be rotated), rash, pruritus

Contraindications
- Hypoglycaemia

Interactions
- *Alcohol*: this enhances the hypoglycaemic effect
- *Beta blockers*: these mask the warning signs of hypoglycaemia; they also enhance the hypoglycaemic effect

Route of administration
- Subcutaneous, IM, IV

Note
- There are five different types of insulin preparations:
  1 Quick-acting insulin analogues (insulin lispro, insulin aspart) – immediate onset, duration of action 4–6 h
  2 Short-acting insulin (soluble insulin) – onset 30 min, duration of action up to 8 h
  3 Intermediate-acting insulin (isophane insulin) – duration of action 14–22 h
  4 Long-acting insulin (e.g. crystalline insulin zinc suspension) – duration of action 36 h; and long-acting insulin analogue (glargine) – duration of action 24 h
  5 Mixed (short-acting with intermediate-acting insulin or analogues)
- Stress, infection, trauma, pregnancy and puberty can increase insulin requirements.
- Insulin promotes the influx of potassium as well as glucose into cells. As a consequence the plasma potassium concentration can drop to dangerously low levels, particularly during insulin treatment of ketoacidosis. In this situation potassium must be replaced intravenously.
- Different regimes are adapted to the individual. Common regimes are a dose of short-acting insulin 15–30 min prior to meals and intermediate-acting insulin at bedtime; or a mixed preparation twice daily (intermediate with short-acting).

Levothyroxine sodium

Class: Thyroid hormone

Indications
- Hypothyroidism

Mechanism of action
- Levothyroxine sodium mimics endogenous thyroxine, thus increasing oxygen consumption of metabolically active tissues.

Adverse effects
- *Rare*: cardiac dysrhythmias, tachycardia, anginal pain, restlessness, sweating, weight loss (all with excessive doses)

Contraindications
- Thyrotoxicosis

Interactions
- *Antiepileptics (carbamazepine, phenytoin)*: these increase the metabolism of levothyroxine
- *Rifampicin*: this increases the metabolism of levothyroxine
- *Warfarin*: levothyroxine increases the effect of warfarin

Route of administration
- Oral

Note
- Plasma TSH levels should be monitored to assess treatment. TSH levels may take 10 weeks to return to normal after optimum thyroxine levels are achieved.
- Levothyroxine should be introduced gradually in patients with IHD, as it can cause excessive cardiac stimulation (consider a pre-therapy ECG).

Related drugs
- Liothyronine sodium (faster acting than levothyroxine sodium)

Metformin

Class: Biguanide

Indications
- Type 2 diabetes mellitus

Mechanism of action
- Exact mechanism is not fully understood.
- Metformin requires the presence of insulin as it is principally an insulin-sensitising agent. It does not influence insulin release.
- Metformin increases peripheral glucose utilisation and decreases gluconeogenesis, possibly through its action on membrane phospholipids.
- It also inhibits glucose absorption from the intestinal lumen.

Adverse effects
- *Common*: anorexia, nausea, vomiting, abdominal pain, diarrhoea
- *Rare*: lactic acidosis (especially in renal impairment), reduced vitamin B_{12} absorption

Contraindications
- Pregnancy
- Breastfeeding
- Use of X-ray contrast
- Use of general anaesthetic
- *Note*: Metformin is also contraindicated in the following conditions, since they predispose to lactic acidosis:
  - Conditions that may cause tissue hypoxia (e.g. respiratory failure, sepsis, severe heart failure)
  - Hepatic or renal impairment
  - Severe dehydration

Interactions
- *Alcohol*: excessive alcohol intake with metformin can predispose to lactic acidosis
- *Corticosteroids*: these antagonise the hypoglycaemic effect of metformin

Route of administration
- Oral

Note
- Metformin does not cause hypoglycaemia, unlike sulphonylureas.
- It is used in type 2 diabetes mellitus patients who do not respond to diet control alone.
- Metformin reduces appetite, thus encouraging weight loss. It is therefore the treatment of choice in obese diabetics.
- Metformin should be stopped prior to receiving iodine-containing X-ray contrast, in order to prevent renal impairment. It should also be stopped prior to general anaesthesia. It can be restarted after the procedure if renal function is normal.

Tamoxifen

Class: Oestrogen receptor antagonist

Indications
- Breast cancer

Mechanism of action
- Exact mechanism is not fully understood.
- Oestrogens are steroid hormones and play a role in proliferation and differentiation of cells. Tamoxifen has both agonist and antagonist action at oestrogen receptors:
    1 It competes with oestradiol at oestrogen receptors in the breast (antagonist action), thereby reducing malignant cell proliferation as well as inducing apoptosis.
    2 It displays oestrogenic effects on the endometrium, bone and blood lipids (agonist action).

Adverse effects
- *Common*: flushing, altered periods, bone pain, nausea, cough, vomiting
- *Rare*: endometrial cancer, thromboembolic events, vaginal bleeding, hypercalcaemia, leukopenia

Contraindications
- Pregnancy
- Caution:
    - History of thromboembolic events

Interactions
- *Warfarin:* tamoxifen increases the anticoagulant effect

Route of administration
- Oral

Note
- A pregnancy test should be performed prior to starting tamoxifen.
- About half of all breast cancer cases in women involve oestrogen receptors, but only about 60% of these will respond to tamoxifen. Tamoxifen has the greatest effect on those tumours that are oestrogen receptor positive. It has a lesser effect on breast cancers with low oestrogen receptor positivity.
- A large number of women develop resistance to tamoxifen after several years of use.
- Tamoxifen is also used in other malignancies, such as brain tumours and malignant melanomas.

SKIN

Management guidelines (pp. 111–112)
Acne
Eczema, atopic
Psoriasis
Rosacea

Individual drugs (pp. 113–116)
Calcitriol; Chlorpheniramine; Dithranol; Isotretinoin

ACNE
- Aim of treatment is to remove the blockage of pilar drainage (comedons) and to treat the infection
- Consider psychological impact on the patient
- Ensure good skin hygiene before initiating treatment
  1 Mild acne:
    - Topical antibiotics – erythromycin, clindamycin
    - Benzoyl peroxide gel
    - Topical isotretinoin (used in comedonal and papulopustular acne)
    - *Note:* Combinations of the above are most effective
  2 Moderate acne:
    - As for mild acne plus oral antibiotics (minocycline), or in females oral oestrogen with cyproterone acetate (antiandrogen)
  3 Severe acne:
    - Oral isotretinoin if the above fails

ATOPIC ECZEMA
- Identify and remove any causative agents (e.g. bleaches, soaps, detergents)
- Topical and systemic agents can be used in various combinations and should be tailored to the individual:
  1 Topical treatment (for mild to moderate eczema):
    - Unscented emollients – used on skin and in bath water (soap substitutes)
    - Coal tar
    - Corticosteroids (ointments for dry chronic eczema; creams for acute weepy eczema)
    - Antibiotics for superimposed infections
  2 Systemic treatment (for moderate to severe eczema):
    - As above plus any of the following:
    - Antihistamines to reduce itching (e.g. chlorpheniramine)
    - UVB phototherapy
    - PUVA radiation
    - Corticosteroids (only used temporarily in severe intractable eczema)

- Consider immunosupressants (ciclosporin or azathioprine) if other treatment options fail
- Antibiotics for superimposed infections
- *Note*: Topical tacrolimus or pimecrolimus can be used if resistant to or unable to tolerate topical steroids

PSORIASIS
- Topical and systemic agents can be used in various combinations and should be tailored to the individual:
  1 Topical treatment (for mild to moderate psoriasis):
    - Emollients
    - Calcitriol or calcipotriol ointment
    - Glucocorticoid ointment (e.g. betamethasone)
    - Coal tar
    - Dithranol cream
    - Tazarotene (a retinoid)
  2 Systemic treatment (for moderate to severe psoriasis):
    - PUVA radiation
    - UVB phototherapy
    - Retinoids (e.g. acitretin)
    - Methotrexate
    - Ciclosporin

ROSACEA
- Avoid precipitants (e.g. hot drinks, alcohol, spicy foods)
- Treatment may be:
  1 Topical – metronidazole, or sodium sulfacetamide with 5% sulphur
  2 Systemic – tetracycline or minocycline, or isotretinoin if antibiotics fail
- Facial flushing can be treated with:
  1 Propranolol or clonidine
  2 Cosmetic camouflage
  3 Laser treatment
- Surgery may be required for complications such as rhinophyma

Calcitriol

Class: Vitamin D analogue

Indications
- Psoriasis (topical use only)
- Hypocalcaemia (e.g. in chronic renal failure, hypoparathyroidism, malabsorption)
- Postmenopausal osteoporosis

Mechanism of action
- Calcitriol is 1,25-dihydroxycholecalciferol, a synthetic hydroxylated form of vitamin D.
- In psoriasis, calcitriol acts by inhibiting fibroblast, lymphocyte and keratinocyte proliferation.
- In hypocalcaemia, calcitriol raises serum calcium by:
  1 stimulating absorption of calcium in the GI tract;
  2 increasing calcium reabsorption in the kidneys, thereby reducing its excretion; and
  3 stimulating calcium release from bones.

Adverse effects
- *Common*: skin irritation and itching with topical use; nausea, vomiting, polyuria, diarrhoea, vertigo and weakness with systemic overdose

Contraindications
- Hypercalcaemia
- Calcifications secondary to metastases

Interactions
- *Thiazide diuretics*: concomitant use increases the risk of hypercalcaemia

Route of administration
- Oral, IV, topical

Note
- Topical calcitriol should be avoided in children and on the face due to irritant effects on the skin.
- Unlike dithranol or tar preparations for psoriasis, topical calcitriol does not smell or stain. It also does not involve the risk of skin atrophy that is seen with topical steroids.
- 90% of the body's vitamin D comes from sunlight exposure, the remaining 10% are dietary (cod liver oil, fatty fish, fortified milk and cereals).
- People not exposed to sunlight are prone to vitamin D deficiency (e.g. housebound elderly). Generally speaking, 15 min of sunlight exposure three times a week will produce adequate vitamin D levels.

Related drugs
- Systemic formulations: alfacalcidol (1 alpha-cholecalciferol), ergocalciferol (vitamin D_2), colecalciferol (vitamin D_3), dihydrotachysterol
- Topical formulations: calcipotriol, tacalcitol

Chlorpheniramine

Class: Histamine 1 receptor antagonist

Indications
- Allergic reactions (e.g. urticaria, hayfever)
- Anaphylaxis

Mechanism of action
- Chlorpheniramine blocks histamine 1 receptors, which are responsible for vasodilatation, oedema and increased capillary permeability. This inhibitory action alleviates symptoms of allergy such as sneezing, itching, swelling and watery eyes.

Adverse effects
- *Common*: antimuscarinic effects (e.g. blurred vision, urinary retention, dry mouth), dizziness, nausea, drowsiness
- *Rare*: palpitations, hepatic dysfunction, tachycardia, paradoxical CNS stimulation

Contraindications
- None
- Caution:
  - Prostatic hypertrophy
  - Glaucoma
  - Urinary retention
  - Hepatic impairment

Interactions
- *TCAs*: muscarinic and sedative effects are enhanced
- *Alcohol*: sedative effects are enhanced

Route of administration
- Oral, IM, subcutaneous, IV

Note
- Chlorpheniramine is less sedating than other 'older' antihistamines in its group. Newer antihistamines are non-sedating (see below).
- Patients should be warned about the possible sedating effects. This is particularly important if driving is involved.
- Drowsiness tends to improve after a few days' use of chlorpheniramine.

Related drugs
- Other sedating antihistamines: brompheniramine, clemastine, cyproheptadine, diphenhydramine, doxylamine, hydroxyzine, promethazine, trimeprazine
- Non-sedating antihistamines: cetirizine, desloratadine, fexofenadine, levocetirizine, loratadine, mizolastine, terfenadine

Dithranol

Class: Anthraquinone derivative

Indications
• Chronic psoriasis

Mechanism of action
• Dithranol is 1,8,9-trihydroxyanthranol, also known as anthralin.
• Dithranol decreases mitotic activity and DNA synthesis in the hyperplastic epidermal layer of the skin. This results in normalisation of epidermal cell proliferation and keratinisation. The end result is inhibition of skin cell growth that occurs in psoriasis.

Adverse effects
• *Common*: irritation of unaffected skin, staining of skin, hair, nails or clothes/bedsheets
• *Rare*: rash

Contraindications
• Acute psoriasis
• Pustular psoriasis

Interactions
• None known

Route of administration
• Topical

Note
• Dithranol should be stopped temporarily in acute flare-ups of psoriasis.
• It should not be used on the face, genitalia or flexures (too irritant).
• To reduce staining, the patient should wear gloves when applying dithranol. When applied at bedtime, old pyjamas should be worn and old bedsheets used.
• Skin irritation caused by accidentally applying dithranol to non-affected skin around a psoriasis plaque can be relieved by applying zinc oxide.
• Treatment with dithranol is usually under the supervision of a dermatologist.

Isotretinoin

Class: Retinoid

Indications
- Acne (especially severe acne and acne not responding to systemic antibiotics)

Mechanism of action
- Exact mechanism is not fully understood.
- It inhibits sebaceous gland function and thereby reduces sebum production.
- Isotretinoin also reduces production of keratin in the outer layer of the skin.
- In addition, isotretinoin has some anti-inflammatory properties.

Adverse effects
- *Common*: dry mucous membranes and skin, photosensitivity, alopecia
- *Rare*: hypertriglyceridaemia, visual disturbances, benign intracranial hypertension, hepatitis, mood changes, hearing impairment, blood disorders

Contraindications
- Pregnancy
- Breastfeeding
- Renal impairment
- Hepatic impairment
- Hypertriglyceridaemia
- Hypervitaminosis A

Interactions
- *Vitamin A*: concomitant use may lead to hypervitaminosis A (stomatitis, dry nose, epistaxis, pruritus)
- *Tetracyclines (doxycycline, minoxycycline, tetracycline):* concomitant use may predispose to benign intracranial hypertension

Route of administration
- Oral, topical

Note
- Isotretinoin should only be prescribed by specialists.
- Regular monitoring of lipids and liver function is essential.
- Dryness of mucous membranes leading to intolerance of contact lenses may occur with retinoid treatment.
- Isotretinoin is teratogenic. Women must be advised to avoid pregnancy whilst taking isotretinoin, and contraception must be used one month before, during and after treatment.

Related drugs
- Acitretin, tretinoin

GENERAL PRINCIPLES OF PAIN CONTROL WITH ANALGESICS
Analgesics are usually divided into two main groups:
1 Primary (non-specific) analgesics,
which can be subdivided into:
  • Simple analgesics (e.g. NSAIDs)
  • Opioid analgesics (e.g. morphine)
2 Secondary (specific) analgesics
  • These medications provide analgesia by removing the cause
  of pain (e.g. GTN spray in angina)

Analgesic ladder
Step 1: non-opioid (e.g. paracetamol, NSAIDs)
Step 2: weak opioid (e.g. co-proxamol, codeine)
Step 3: strong opioid (e.g. morphine, fentanyl)
• Inadequate analgesia requires a move to the next step rather
than to another drug of similar efficacy

ALTERNATIVE METHODS OF PAIN CONTROL
• Psychological care (e.g. explanation of pain, reassurance)
• Hot or cold applications (e.g. hot water bottle, ice pack)
• Immobilisation with collars, splints, corsets, etc.
• Acupuncture
• TENS
• Nerve block using local anaesthetic

BONE PAIN
• Treat any underlying cause
• Administer an NSAID (e.g. diclofenac)
• Radiotherapy is effective in metastatic bone pain
• Calcitonin, corticosteroids or opioids may also be used

MUSCLE SPASM PAIN
- Treat any underlying cause
- **Smooth muscle spasm:**
  - Typically experienced in renal colic or intestinal colic
  - Give hyoscine butylbromide, a smooth muscle relaxant
  - Stronger analgesia (e.g. opioids) may be required
- **Skeletal muscle spasm:**
  - May be experienced in multiple sclerosis, spinal cord injury or other trauma
  - The following agents may be used:
    1 Baclofen, a skeletal muscle relaxant that acts centrally and on the spinal cord
    2 Diazepam, which acts on GABA receptors in the CNS
    3 Dantrolene, which acts peripherally on skeletal muscle
  - *Note*: Above medications should not be used for muscular spasm caused by minor injuries
- **Nocturnal leg cramps:**
  - Quinine can be used long-term. It reduces the frequency of cramps by roughly 25%
  - Effect may not be apparent for up to 4 weeks
  - Treatment should be interrupted every 3 months to assess the need for continuing therapy

NEUROPATHIC PAIN
- Treat initially with a TCA (e.g. amitriptyline)
- Gabapentin, carbamazepine, capsaicin or phenytoin may be used if 1st line treatment has failed
- Opioids are only partially effective in neuropathic pain. Consider these when other treatment options have failed.
- TENS may be effective in some patients
- Surgery may be an option in some cases

Drug classes

NON-STEROIDAL ANTI-INFLAMMATORY DRUGS
Types of NSAIDs
1 Salicylic acids: aspirin
2 Propionic acids: ibuprofen, naproxen
3 Acetic acids: indometacin
4 Fenemates: mefenamic acid
5 Pyrazolones: phenylbutazone
6 Phenylacetic acids: diclofenac
7 Oxicams: meloxicam, piroxicam, tenoxicam
8 COX-2 inhibitors: celecoxib, etodolac, etoricoxib, valdecoxib

Indications
- Inflammatory diseases (e.g. rheumatoid arthritis)

- Pain (especially musculoskeletal pain)
- Perioperative analgesia (alongside opioids and local anaesthetics – concept known as 'balanced analgesia')
- Pyrexia

Mechanism of action
- NSAIDs act through reversible inhibition of COX-1 and COX-2, which results in decreased conversion of arachidonic acid to prostaglandins.
- Aspirin differs in the fact that it irreversibly inhibits COX-1 and COX-2. It also has an antiplatelet effect.
- COX-2 inhibitors specifically target COX-2.
- The desired pharmacological effects of NSAIDs are thought to be due to the inhibition of COX-2.

Adverse effects
- These are mainly related to the inhibition of COX-1 and include:
  - GI disturbances (peptic ulcer, gastritis)
  - Bleeding (with aspirin)
  - Bronchoconstriction
  - Renal impairment

OPIOID ANALGESICS
Indications
- Pain is the main indication (morphine or diamorphine are most commonly used in severe pain)
- Other uses:
  - Acute pulmonary oedema secondary to heart failure (morphine or diamorphine)
  - Diarrhoea (codeine)
  - Cough (codeine or dihydrocodeine)
- Methadone is used to prevent withdrawal symptoms in opioid abusers

Mechanism of action
- Opioid analgesics mimic endogenous opioids by acting on μ, δ and κ opioid receptors in the spinal cord and in areas of the brainstem that are rich in naturally occurring opioids.
  1 Full agonists: codeine, dextropropoxyphene, diamorphine, dihydrocodeine, fentanyl, morphine, pethidine
  2 Partial agonists: buprenorphine, pentazocine, tramadol

Adverse effects
- Respiratory depression (with high doses)
- Constipation
- Nausea and vomiting
- Dependence and tolerance (dependence very rarely occurs when used correctly for pain)

Opioid antagonists

- These are used to reverse severe or unwanted opioid effects, which usually occur after overdose:
  - Naloxone (rapidly acting)
  - Naltrexone (longer duration of action)

Note

- Codeine is commonly used as a weaker alternative to morphine.
- Opioid antagonists or abrupt withdrawal of an opioid can precipitate a withdrawal syndrome. This typically becomes evident after about 12 h. It can include symptoms such as yawning, sweating and rhinorrhoea, followed by irritability, insomnia, tremor and gooseflesh ('cold turkey' effect). Symptoms reach a peak 2–3 days after withdrawal and recede after about 1 week. Diarrhoea, vomiting and abdominal cramps may also occur.

Co-proxamol

Class: Compound analgesic (paracetamol +
dextropropoxyphene)

Indications
  • Moderate pain
Mechanism of action
  • The paracetamol component inhibits production of
  chemical mediators that cause pain (see Paracetamol).
  • The dextropropoxyphene component acts by binding to
  opioid receptors in the CNS to decrease pain (see Morphine).
Adverse effects
  • *Common*: nausea, vomiting, constipation, drowsiness
  • *Rare*: rash, euphoria
Contraindications
  • None
  • Caution:
    • Asthma
    • Chronic respiratory disease
    • Elderly
    • Therapy with hepatic enzyme-inducing drugs (e.g.
    anticonvulsants, alcohol)
Interactions
  • See, Morphine, Paracetamol (pp. 123 and 124)
Route of administration
  • Oral
Note
  • If co-proxamol is prescribed long-term, tolerance and
  dependence may develop due to the dextropropoxyphene
  component.
  • Co-proxamol overdose can be hazardous as
  dextropropoxyphene may cause respiratory depression and
  paracetamol may lead to liver damage.
  • There is no evidence that co-proxamol is superior to
  paracetamol in short-term use.
Related drugs
  • Co-codamol (paracetamol + codeine phosphate),
  co-dydramol (paracetamol + dihydrocodeine)

Diclofenac

Class: Non-steroidal anti-inflammatory drug

Indications
- Musculoskeletal and postoperative pain
- Prophylaxis of eye inflammation post cataract surgery (topical application)
- Actinic keratosis (topical application)

Mechanism of action
- Diclofenac is a potent inhibitor of enzymes COX-1 and COX-2. This leads to inhibition of prostaglandin synthesis and hence to:

  1 a decrease in vascular permeability and vasodilatation (anti-inflammatory effect);

  2 a decrease in sensitisation of pain afferents (analgesic effect); and

  3 a decrease in the effect of prostaglandins on the hypothalamus (antipyretic effect).

Adverse effects
- *Common*: nausea, diarrhoea, epigastric discomfort, prolonged bleeding time
- *Rare*: gluteal abscess (when injected IM), peptic ulceration and bleeding, bronchospasm, renal failure, fluid retention

Contraindications
- Previous or current peptic ulceration
- Caution:
  - Renal and hepatic impairment
  - Asthma
  - Coagulation defects
  - Pregnancy and breastfeeding

Interactions
- *Corticosteroids*: increased risk of peptic ulceration when diclofenac is given with corticosteroids

Route of administration
- IM, IV, oral, rectal, topical

Note
- Clinically diclofenac is used in postoperative pain, acute gout, other musculoskeletal pain, and ureteric colic.
- Diclofenac does not cause respiratory depression, dependence or impaired GI motility.
- Full analgesic effect of diclofenac is normally achieved after 1 week of therapy. It may take up to 3 weeks to achieve full anti-inflammatory effect.
- IM or rectal diclofenac has a comparable effect to pethidine in the management of ureteric colic.
- Diclofenac topical gel is effective in the treatment of actinic keratosis. In this instance it should be continued for 2–3 months.

Morphine

Class: Opioid analgesic

Indications
- Severe pain (e.g. MI, perioperative analgesia, pain in terminal illness)
- Acute pulmonary oedema secondary to heart failure
- Intractable cough in terminal care

Mechanism of action
- Morphine mimics endogenous opioids by acting on μ, δ and κ opioid receptors in the spinal cord and in areas of the brainstem that are rich in naturally occuring opioids.
- In MI and pulmonary oedema, morphine reduces preload by dilating large veins

Adverse effects
- *Common*: nausea, vomiting, drowsiness, constipation; respiratory depression and hypotension with larger doses
- *Rare*: hallucinations, difficulty with micturition, dry mouth, urticaria, biliary spasm, mood changes

Contraindications
- Acute respiratory depression
- Raised intracranial pressure (morphine may interfere with neurological assessment)
- Head injury (morphine may interfere with neurological assessment)
- Phaeochromocytoma
- Acute alcohol intoxication
- Paralytic ileus

Interactions
- *Alcohol*: this enhances the sedative and hypotensive effects of morphine
- *Hypnotics*: these enhance the sedative and hypotensive effects of morphine

Route of administration
- IM, IV, oral, rectal, subcutaneous

Note
- The effects of morphine can be reversed with naloxone, a rapidly acting opioid antagonist.
- Tolerance to morphine begins to emerge after about 2 weeks of continuous administration. Subsequently, the dose should be increased.
- Dependence on morphine develops gradually. It is very uncommon when used to treat pain.
- Abrupt withdrawal of morphine results in a withdrawal syndrome (myalgia, sweating, yawning).

Related drugs
- Codeine, dextropropoxyphene, diamorphine, fentanyl, methadone, pethidine

Paracetamol

Class: Non-opioid analgesic and antipyretic

Indications
- Mild to moderate pain
- Pyrexia

Mechanism of action
- Paracetamol is a weak inhibitor of both COX-1 and COX-2, which are responsible for the production of prostaglandins and thromboxane.
- Paracetamol may also act through selective inhibition of COX-3, a more recently discovered enzyme found in the brain and spinal cord.
- It is believed that these actions result in analgesic and antipyretic effects of paracetamol without GI adverse effects.

Adverse effects
- *Rare*: rash, blood dyscrasias; hepatic necrosis and renal failure in overdose

Contraindications
- None
- Caution:
  - Hepatic impairment
  - Renal impairment
  - Chronic alcohol abuse

Interactions
- No serious interactions

Route of administration
- Oral, rectal

Note
- Paracetamol has similar analgesic efficacy to aspirin. As paracetamol does not cause gastric irritation it is preferred to aspirin for pain relief, especially in the elderly.
- Paracetamol is commonly used in children as it is not associated with Reye's syndrome (unlike aspirin).
- Paracetamol is effective in musculoskeletal pain. Opioids are preferred in visceral pain.
- Toxic metabolites of paracetamol are generated more rapidly when administered with drugs that induce hepatic enzymes (e.g. rifampicin).
- *N*-acetylcysteine is an effective antidote in paracetamol overdose (see p. 186).
- Paracetamol does not exert any antiplatelet action (unlike aspirin).

Pethidine

Class: Opioid analgesic

Indications
- Moderate to severe pain (e.g. perioperatively, labour)

Mechanism of action
- Pethidine acts by stimulating opioid μ, δ and κ receptors in the spinal cord and in areas of the brainstem that are rich in naturally occurring opioids.
- It creates a sense of euphoria, which contributes to the analgesic effect by reducing anxiety and stress.

Adverse effects
- *Common*: nausea, vomiting, constipation, drowsiness, dizziness, confusion
- *Rare*: shortness of breath, convulsions in overdose

Contraindications
- Severe renal impairment
- Respiratory failure
- Alcoholism
- Concomitant use of MAOIs

Interactions
- *Cimetidine*: this inhibits metabolism of pethidine and thus increases its plasma concentration
- *MAOIs*: these given with pethidine can cause CNS excitation or CNS depression

Route of administration
- Oral, IM, IV, subcutaneous

Note
- Owing to its lipid-solubility, pethidine has a rapid onset of action. It is a less potent analgesic than morphine.
- Pethidine can be used in labour, as adverse effects on the baby are less pronounced than with other opioids (due to its short half-life of 2–4 h), and also because it does not inhibit uterine contractions. Pethidine may, however, cause respiratory depression in the neonate if given to the labouring mother.
- Larger doses of pethidine are required if given orally due to extensive first-pass metabolism.
- Unlike morphine, pethidine does not cause pupillary constriction in overdose. Naloxone is an effective antidote in pethidine overdose.
- Pethidine is less constipating than morphine.
- Norpethidine, a metabolite of pethidine, may accumulate and cause convulsions by stimulating the CNS. This is more likely in renal impairment.

Related drugs
- Diamorphine, fentanyl, methadone, morphine

Types of antibiotics (pp. 127–131)
Antibacterials
Antifungals
Antivirals

Management guidelines (pp. 131–136)
Cellulitis
Conjunctivitis
Endocarditis
  infective
Erysipelas
Human immunodeficiency virus
Impetigo
Meningitis
  bacterial
  viral
Necrotising fasciitis
Otitis media
Pelvic infection (pelvic inflammatory disease)
Pneumonia
Septicaemia
Tonsillitis/Throat infections
Tuberculosis
Urinary tract infections
  cystitis
  pyelonephritis
  urethritis

Individual drugs (pp. 137–152)
Aciclovir; Amoxicillin; Benzylpenicillin; Cefuroxime;
Chloramphenicol; Ciprofloxacin; Clotrimazole;
Erythromycin; Flucloxacillin; Gentamicin; Metronidazole;
Rifampicin; Tetracycline; Trimethoprim; Vancomycin;
Zidovudine

ANTIBACTERIALS
Antibacterial agents work by acting on microbial
components that are either absent or radically different in
human cells (i.e. selective toxicity). There are three main
mechanisms by which they arrest microbial growth, as detailed
below.
1 *Inhibition of cell wall synthesis*
  • Penicillins
    • Benzylpenicillin (penicillin G), phenoxymethylpenicillin
      (penicillin V)
    • Broad-spectrum penicillins: amoxicillin, ampicillin

- Antipseudomonal penicillins: azlocillin, piperacillin, ticarcillin
- Beta-lactamase resisitant penicillins: cloxacillin, dicloxacillin, flucloxacillin
- Mecillinams
  - Pivmecillinam
- Cephalosporins
  - *1st generation*: cefazolin, cefradine, cefaclor, cefadroxil, cefalexin
  - *2nd generation*: cefuroxime, cefamandole
  - *3rd generation*: cefodizime, cefotaxime, ceftazidime, ceftizoxine, ceftriaxone, cefixime, ceftibuten, cefpodoxim proxetil
  - *4th generation*: cefepime, cefpirome
  - Antipseudomonal cephalosporins: cefepime, ceftazidime
- Glycopeptides
  - Teicoplanin, vancomicin
- Carbapenems
  - Ertapenem, imipenem, meropenem
- Monobactams
  - Aztreonam

2 *Inhibition of nucleic acid synthesis*
- Quinolones
  - Cinoxacin, ciprofloxacin, gatifloxacin, levofloxacin, moxifloxacin, nalidixic acid, norfloxacin, ofloxacin
- Trimethoprim
- Sulphonamides
  - Sulphamethoxazole
- Nitroimidazoles
  - Metronidazole, ornidazole, tinidazole
- Nitrofurantoin
- Rifampicin

3 *Inhibition of protein synthesis*
- (a) By acting on the 30S bacterial ribosomal subunit:
  - Aminoglycosides
    - Amikacin, gentamicin, kanamicin, neomicin, netilmicin, tobramicin, streptomicin
  - Tetracyclines
    - Doxycycline, lymecycline, minocycline, oxytetracycline, tetracycline
- (b) By acting on the 50S bacterial ribosomal subunit:
  - Macrolides
  - Azithromicin, clarithromicin, erythromicin, roxithromicin, telithromicin, spiramicin
  - Oxazolidinones
  - Linezolid
  - Streptogramins
  - Quinupristin-dalfopristin
  - Clindamicin

- Chloramphenicol
- Fusidic acid

The following tables show some common pathogens and antibiotics that can be used to treat them. It should be noted that resistance to many antibiotics is emerging and the regimens shown here are subject to change.

Pathogen	Treatment of choice
Anaerobes	Metronidazole
Bordetella pertussis	Erythromicin
Campylobacter spp.	Ciprofloxacin or erythromicin
Chlamydia trachomatis	Doxycycline
Clostridium difficile	Stop any antibiotics ± give oral metronidazole or oral vancomicin
Corynebacterium diphtheriae	Erythromicin
Enterococcus spp.	Amoxicillin/ ampicillin ± gentamicin
Escherichia coli	Trimethoprim for cystitis Ceftriaxone/gentamicin for serious infections
Giardia lamblia	Metronidazole
Haemophilus influenzae	Cefotaxime or co-amoxiclav
Legionella pneumophila	Erythromicin
Listeria monocytogenes	Ampicillin + gentamicin
Mycobacterium tuberculosis	Rifampicin + isoniazid + pyrazinamide (± ethambutol)
Mycoplasma pneumoniae	Erythromicin or tetracycline
Neisseria gonorrhoea	Ceftriaxone or ciprofloxacin
Neisseria meningitidis	Any beta-lactam (ceftriaxone preferred)
Pseudomonas aeruginosa	Aminoglycoside + antipseudomonal penicillin
Salmonella spp.	Ciprofloxacin
Shigella dysenteriae	Ciprofloxacin
Staphylococcus spp.	Flucloxacillin if not methicillin-resistant, vancomicin for MRSA
Streptococcus spp.	Penicillin or cephalosporin
Vibrio cholerae	Tetracycline

ANTIFUNGALS
Fungal infections (termed mycoses) are difficult to treat. Being eukaryotic, their metabolic pathways are more similar to mammalian cells and therefore present fewer targets for

chemotherapy. They usually involve the skin, nails or mucous membranes. Systemic fungal infections usually occur in immunocompromised individuals. There are four main classes of antifungal drugs:

1 Imidazoles – These act by inhibiting synthesis of lipids in the fungal cell membrane (e.g. clotrimazole, miconazole, ketoconazole)

2 Polyenes – These act by forming pores in the fungal membrane, leading to cell death (e.g. amphotericin, nystatin)

3 Triazoles – These act by a mechanism similar to the imidazoles (e.g. fluconazole, itraconazole)

4 Others – These include flucytosine, griseofulvin and terbinafine

Fungus	Treatment of choice
Aspergillus spp.	Amphotericin
Blastomyces spp.	Itraconazole
Candida spp.	Local therapy: nystatin/ clotrimazole
	Systemic therapy: fluconazole/ amphotericin
Coccidioides spp.	Amphotericin
Cryptococcus neoformans	Amphotericin/fluconazole
Histoplasma capsulatum	Amphotericin/itraconazole
Malassezia furfur (Pityriasis versicolor)	Local therapy: terbinafine
	Systemic therapy: Itraconazole
Paracoccidioides spp.	Itraconazole
Dermatophytes (epidermophyton, microsporum, trichophyton)	Griseofulvin/imidazoles

ANTIVIRALS

• Viruses, which live and replicate inside human cells, make use of the metabolic pathways of the host cell. It is thus very difficult to direct treatment selectively against the virus without in some way adversely affecting the patient.

• There are three general mechanisms by which antiviral agents work:

1 Inhibition of viral nucleic acid synthesis (e.g. aciclovir, foscarnet, ganciclovir, ribavirin, zidovudine)

2 Immunomodulatory action (e.g. immunoglobulins, interferons)

3 Inhibition of specific viral targets (e.g. amantadine, ritonavir, oseltamivir, pleconaril, zanamivir)

Virus	Treatment of choice
Cytomegalovirus	Ganciclovir
Hepatitis B	Interferon alpha 2a and lamivudine
Hepatitis C	Interferon alpha 2a and ribavirin
Hepatitis D	Treat hepatitis B
Herpes simplex	Aciclovir
Human immunodeficiency virus	Highly active antiretroviral therapy (HAART) – see pp. 132–133
Influenza A	Oseltamivir/zanamivir
Respiratory syncitial virus	Consider nebulised ribavirin
Varicella zoster	Aciclovir (IV route), valaciclovir (oral route)

Management guidelines

CELLULITIS
• Cellulitis is usually caused by a combination of staphylococci and Group A streptococci.
• Treat systemically with co-amoxiclav to cover both above-mentioned organisms.
• Depending on the site (e.g. diabetic foot), broad-spectrum cover may be required (e.g. gentamicin with co-amoxiclav).

CONJUNCTIVITIS (INFECTIVE)
• Usually caused by *Staphylococcus aureus*, *Streptococcus pneumoniae*, *Haemophilus influenzae* or adenoviruses.
• Most cases are self-resolving. If treatment is desired, give chloramphenicol eye drops or ointment (this covers all the aforementioned pathogens except adenovirus, for which there is no treatment available). Remember to treat both eyes (cross-infection is common).
• In allergic conjunctivitis, give sodium cromoglycate or antihistamine eye drops.

INFECTIVE ENDOCARDITIS
• Detailed guidelines exist and consultation with a cardiologist or infectious disease specialist is recommended.

Prophylaxis of infective endocarditis
• Prophylaxis is necessary in patients with cardiac abnormalities (e.g. congenital defects, valvular heart disease, artificial heart valves) and other high-risk groups (e.g. previous infective endocarditis) undergoing the following:
  1 Dental procedures under local or no anaesthetic:
    • Give oral amoxicillin 1 h before the dental procedure (oral clindamycin if allergic to penicillin or if penicillin was given in the past month)
    • Add gentamicin if the patient has had previous endocarditis
  2 Surgery or GI/urinary tract instrumentation:
    • Give IV amoxicillin + IV gentamicin

Treatment of infective endocarditis
• Treatment depends on organism susceptibility and usually lasts for about 2–4 weeks
• Typical regimens are:
  • Streptococcal endocarditis: give IV benzylpenicillin/ceftriaxone ± IV gentamicin
  • Staphylococcal endocarditis: give IV flucloxacillin/vancomicin ± IV gentamicin
  • Enterococcal endocarditis: give IV amoxicillin ± IV gentamicin
• If no response to antibiotics, consider surgery (valve replacement)

ERYSIPELAS
• Erysipelas is usually caused by Group A streptococci.
• Treat systemically with penicillin.

HUMAN IMMUNODEFICIENCY VIRUS
• There is no cure for HIV, but the aim of treatment is to reduce viral load and thereby increase the CD4 cell count (T_4 'helper' cells).
• Treatment for HIV must be under specialist supervision or undertaken by a doctor with experience in the field.
• Apart from antiretroviral therapy, the patient may also be on treatment for opportunistic infections such as CMV retinitis or *Pneumocystis carinii* pneumonia.
• Three categories of antiretroviral agents used in HIV are available:
  1 nucleoside analogue reverse transcriptase inhibitors (NRTIs): abacavir, didanosine, lamivudine, stavudine, tenofovir disoproxil, zalcitabine, zidovudine
  2 non-nucleoside reverse transcriptase inhibitors (non-NRTIs): efavirenz, nevirapine
  3 protease inhibitors: amprenavir, indinavir, nelfinavir, ritonavir, saquinavir

- Treatment is usually two NRTIs with a protease inhibitor, or two NRTIs with a non-NRTI. However, these regimes are subject to frequent updates and changes.

IMPETIGO
- Impetigo is usually caused by staphylococci and Group A streptococci.
- For limited skin involvement, give topical fusidic acid or mupirocin.
- For more extensive skin involvement, give oral flucloxacillin or erythromycin.

BACTERIAL MENINGITIS
Neonates
- Most likely organisms are:
  - Group B streptococci – treat with IV benzylpenicillin
  - *Escherichia coli* – treat with IV cefotaxime
  - *Listeria monocytogenes* – treat with IV ampicillin + IV gentamicin
- Blind therapy – IV penicillin + IV gentamicin

Infant/toddler
- Most likely organisms are:
  - *Neisseria meningitidis* – treat with IV cefotaxime
  - *Streptococcus pneumoniae* – treat with IV cefotaxime
  - *Haemophilus influenzae* – treat with IV cefotaxime (incidence decreasing due to Hib vaccine)
- Blind therapy – IV cefotaxime

From age 4 onwards
- Most likely organisms are:
  - *Neisseria meningitidis* – treat with IV cefotaxime
  - *Streptococcus pneumoniae* – treat with IV cefotaxime
- Blind therapy – IV cefotaxime

Note
- IV fluids may be given if required.
- Dexamethasone may be given to decrease the risk of complications of meningitis in children (e.g. deafness, cerebral oedema).
- Oral rifampicin is given to close contacts such as family members for a period of 48 h to prevent spread of meningitis caused by *Neisseria meningitidis* or *Haemophilus influenzae*.
- Meningococcal meningitis is not to be confused with meningococcal septicaemia. Both are medical emergencies. If suspected, IV cefotaxime (or IM benzylpenicillin if in the

community) should be given immediately *before* any
investigations are undertaken.

VIRAL MENINGITIS
• Viruses cause 'aseptic' meningitis, as opposed to the
'pyogenic' meningitis caused by bacteria such as *Neisseria
meningitidis*. Causative agents of viral meningitis include
mumps, herpes and enteroviruses.
• Treatment is supportive (e.g. bed rest, analgesia) as viral
meningitis is self-limiting.

NECROTISING FASCIITIS
• Causative agents are usually multiple, including Group A
streptococci. Anaerobes are frequently involved due to the
hypoxic tissue damage that occurs.
• Broad-spectrum antibiotics are the key. Treat systemically
with penicillin and clindamicin, and add gentamicin if
polymicrobial. Alternatively, give gentamicin and co-
amoxiclav.
• Surgical debridement is usually required.
• Hyperbaric oxygen may be useful.

OTITIS MEDIA
• Otitis media is caused by bacteria or viruses. Common
bacterial organisms are S*treptococcus pneumoniae* and
Haemophilus influenzae.
• Most cases of acute otitis media are self-resolving, but
decongestants may be useful and oral co-amoxiclav can be
given if desired (in severe cases given IV).
• In chronic otitis media consider myringotomy and grommet
insertion (remember that 80% of chronic otitis media in
children resolve without treatment).

PELVIC INFECTION (PELVIC INFLAMMATORY DISEASE)
• Commonest cause is *Chlamydia trachomatis* followed by
Neisseria gonorrhoeae.
• Treat promptly for 10–14 days to prevent complications such
as infertility and ectopic pregnancies: oral ofloxacin with
metronidazole, or oral co-amoxiclav with doxycycline
• Remove IUCD if present.
• Give analgesia if required (many patients are asymptomatic).
• Consider laparoscopy if antibiotics are ineffective (diagnosis
of pelvic infection may be incorrect).
• Recommend barrier contraception or abstinence until
recovery is made to prevent spread of the infection.
• Contact screening is recommended.

PNEUMONIA
Principles of management
- Bed rest
- Pain relief ± antiemetic
- Oral/IV fluids
- High-flow oxygen if required
- Chest physiotherapy
- IV antibiotics (see below) after relevant investigations including blood and sputum cultures

Community-acquired pneumonia
- Mostly caused by *Streptococcus pneumoniae*, followed by *Mycoplasma pneumoniae*
- Treat with amoxicillin (plus erythromicin in severe cases)

Hospital-acquired pneumonia
- Often caused by *Pseudomonas aeruginosa*, *Klebsiella*, *Staphylococcus aureus*, *Escherichia coli*
- Treatment is usually a broad-spectrum cephalosporin such as ceftazidime (plus an aminoglycoside in severe cases)

Atypical pneumonia
- Mostly caused by *Mycoplasma pneumoniae*, *Chlamydia* spp., *Coxiella burnetii* and *Legionella* spp. infections
- Treat with erythromycin or tetracycline

SEPTICAEMIA
- Rehydrate
- Take blood, urine, sputum and wound cultures before starting antibiotic therapy
- Choice of antibiotic depends on the likely source: flucloxacillin for *Staphylococcus aureus*, gentamicin for Gram-negatives (e.g. UTI), cephalosporin or penicillin for Gram-positives, and metronidazole if there are abdominal signs
- When laboratory results are available, adapt antibiotic therapy if necessary
- Inotropes (e.g. dobutamine) may be required if haemodynamically compromised
- Investigate the source of sepsis and treat accordingly

TONSILLITIS/THROAT INFECTIONS
- More than half of tonsillitis cases are due to viral infection and therefore not amenable to antibiotic treatment. If you do decide to give an antibiotic, penicillin is the agent of choice since the most common bacterial cause is *Streptococcus pyogenes*.
- One of the aims of treating tonsillitis is to prevent rheumatic fever

- Remember that amoxicillin causes a rash if given to patients with infectious mononucleosis (i.e. EBV infection)

TUBERCULOSIS
Phase 1: rifampicin + isoniazid + pyrazinamide for 2 months
Phase 2: rifampicin + isoniazid for 4 months
- In cases of suspected isoniazid resistance, ethambutol may be given
- Give pyridoxine (vitamin B_6) throughout treatment as isoniazid can cause vitamin B_6 deficiency

URINARY TRACT INFECTIONS
- UTIs can be divided into infections of the kidney (pyelonephritis), bladder (cystitis) and urethra (urethritis)
- The commonest cause is *Escherichia coli*

Principles of management
- Increase fluid intake
- Analgesia
- Antibiotics (see below)

Children
- Management should be initiated in consultation with a paediatrician
- The child should be investigated for any underlying structural abnormalities (e.g. ureteric obstruction) and vesicoureteric reflux whilst maintaining therapy with oral trimethoprim

Adults
- Pyelonephritis – IV gentamicin
- Cystitis – oral trimethoprim (if pregnant, give oral amoxicillin or nitrofurantoin)
- Urethritis – usually chlamydial (treat with oral azithromycin or tetracycline); if gonococcal, treat with oral ciprofloxacin or IM ceftriaxone

Note
- Cystitis is the most common form of UTI and can usually be treated with a single dose or a short course of antibiotic.
- Males who present with a first episode of cystitis or pyelonephritis should be investigated for underlying pathology (e.g. obstruction due to prostate enlargement or renal calculi).

Aciclovir

Class: Antiviral agent

Indications
- Infections caused by alpha herpes viruses (herpes simplex types 1 and 2, varicella zoster virus)

Mechanism of action
- Aciclovir is selectively taken up by virus-infected cells. It is preferentially phosphorylated by herpes virus–encoded thymidine kinase to aciclovir monophosphate. This is then converted to aciclovir triphosphate by cellular phosphokinases. Aciclovir triphosphate is incorporated into herpes DNA and acts as a chain terminator.

Adverse effects
- *Rare*: rash (topical lotion); nausea, vomiting, headache (oral route); renal impairment (if given too quickly IV); confusion, hallucinations (IV route); inflammation at the drip site (if there is leakage into tissues)

Contraindications
- None
- Caution:
  - Pregnancy and breastfeeding

Interactions
- *Probenecid*: this increases the plasma concentration of aciclovir by decreasing its excretion (this does not apply to topical aciclovir preparations)

Route of administration
- Oral, topical, IV

Note
- Aciclovir is prescribed for herpes simplex types 1 and 2 infections (genital herpes, cold sores, encephalitis, eye infections). It is also used to treat shingles and chickenpox, both caused by varicella zoster virus.
- If encephalitis is suspected, IV aciclovir should be given immediately.
- Ganciclovir is more effective than aciclovir in the treatment of CMV and EBV infections (but is also more toxic).
- In aciclovir resistance, foscarnet or cidofovir should be used.

Related drugs
- Famciclovir, ganciclovir, penciclovir, valaciclovir

Amoxicillin

Class: Beta-lactam antibiotic

Indications
- Wide range of infections caused by Gram-positive (e.g. *Streptococcus* spp., *Staphylococcus* spp.) and Gram-negative (e.g. *Haemophilus influenzae*) bacteria
- Part of *Helicobacter pylori* eradication therapy
- Prophylaxis of infectious endocarditis prior to dental/surgical procedures

Mechanism of action
- Amoxicillin is a broad-spectrum bactericidal antibiotic.
- It inhibits bacterial cell wall synthesis by preventing formation of cross-links between peptidoglycan chains that constitute the bacterial cell wall.

Adverse effects
- *Common*: rash, diarrhoea, nausea, vomiting, candida vaginitis
- *Rare*: anaphylaxis, antibiotic-associated colitis

Contraindications
- Penicillin hypersensitivity

Interactions
- *COC pill*: amoxicillin may reduce the effectiveness of the pill
- *Probenecid*: this decreases the excretion of amoxicillin

Route of administration
- Oral, IM, IV

Note
- Certain strains of bacteria produce the enzyme beta-lactamase, which inactivates amoxicillin. In order to prevent this inactivation, amoxicillin can be usefully combined with clavulanic acid (known as co-amoxiclav).
- Amoxicillin characteristically causes a rash if given to patients with infectious mononucleosis.
- Patients also taking the COC pill should be advised to take other contraceptive precautions.

Related drugs
- Ampicillin (less well absorbed orally)

Benzylpenicillin (penicillin G)

Class: Beta-lactam antibiotic

Indications
- Infections caused by *Streptococcus* spp., *Neisseria meningitidis* and *Neisseria gonorrhoeae*
- Also used in infections caused by *Treponema pallidum*, *Corynebacterium diphtheriae*, *Clostridium tetani*, *Bacillus anthracis*, *Leptospira* spp. and other susceptible organisms

Mechanism of action
- Benzylpenicillin is a bactericidal antibiotic.
- It inhibits bacterial cell wall synthesis by preventing formation of cross-links between peptidoglycan chains that constitute the bacterial cell wall.

Adverse effects
- *Common*: rash, diarrhoea
- *Rare*: anaphylaxis; bone marrow suppression and convulsions in high doses, encephalopathy, cardiac dysrhythmias

Contraindications
- Penicillin hypersensitivity

Interactions
- *Probenecid*: this decreases the excretion of benzylpenicillin (a useful interaction that allows dose reduction of penicillin)

Route of administration
- IV, IM

Note
- Benzylpenicillin is inactivated by the enzyme beta-lactamase, which is produced by many organisms (e.g. most *Staphylococcus* spp., some strains of *Escherichia coli* and *Pseudomonas*). These organisms can be treated with beta-lactamase-resistant penicillins or antipseudomonal penicillins.
- In cases of penicillin allergy erythromycin can be given.
- 1–10% of patients given a penicillin experience an allergic reaction. Less than 0.05% suffer an anaphylaxis. These hypersensitivity reactions are triggered by the breakdown products of penicillin.

Related drugs
- Penicillin V (oral equivalent of benzylpenicillin)

Cefuroxime

Class: 2nd generation cephalosporin (beta-lactam antibiotic)

Indications
- Infections caused by Gram-positive (e.g. *Streptococcus* spp., *Staphylococcus* spp.) and Gram-negative bacteria (e.g. *Escherichia coli, Haemophilus influenzae*)

Mechanism of action
- Cefuroxime inhibits bacterial cell wall synthesis by preventing formation of cross-links between peptidoglycan chains that constitute the bacterial cell wall.

Adverse effects
- *Common*: diarrhoea, thrombophlebitis (at the site of IV injection)
- *Rare*: haemorrhage, hypersensitivity, nausea, vomiting, antibiotic-associated colitis

Contraindications
- Hypersensitivity
- Porphyria
- Caution:
  - Penicillin allergy (see below)

Interactions
- *Probenecid*: this increases the plasma concentration of cefuroxime by decreasing its excretion
- *Warfarin*: cefuroxime may enhance the anticoagulant effect of warfarin

Route of administration
- Oral, IM, IV, eye drops

Note
- Currently there are four generations of cephalosporins available (see p. 128)
- 1st and 2nd generation cephalosporins are used against both Gram-negative and Gram-positive organisms.
- 3rd generation cephalosporins are less toxic, more efficacious and more specific towards Gram-negative organisms.
- 4th generation cephalosporins have increased antistaphylococcal activity and are more active against enterobacteriaceae than 3rd generation cephalosporins.
- About 10% of patients who are allergic to penicillin will have an allergic reaction to cephalosporins. This is due to a similar chemical structure.

Related drugs
- Cefamandole

Chloramphenicol

Class: Antibacterial agent

Indications
- Gram-positive and Gram-negative bacterial infections, including anaerobes
- *Rickettsia, Mycoplasma* and *Chlamydia* spp. infections

Mechanism of action
- Chloramphenicol is a bacteriostatic antibiotic.
- It binds to the 50S subunit of the bacterial ribosome and thereby inhibits protein synthesis. This prevents bacterial reproduction.

Adverse effects
- *Common*: nausea, diarrhoea, anorexia
- *Rare*: reversible or irreversible aplastic anaemia, optic and peripheral neuritis, grey baby syndrome in neonates, urticaria

Contraindications
- Pregnancy
- Breastfeeding
- Porphyria

Interactions
- *Phenytoin:* risk of phenytoin toxicity
- *Warfarin*: increased effect of warfarin

Route of administration
- Oral, IV, topical

Note
- Clinically chloramphenicol is used in otitis externa, typhoid fever and conjunctivitis. It is also used in bacterial meningitis if allergic to penicillin or cephalosporins.
- Chloramphenicol should be used as a 2nd line antibiotic due to its potentially lethal adverse effects (aplastic anaemia).
- Aplastic anaemia may occur during or after chloramphenicol treatment. If occurring after, it is usually irreversible.
- Patients should not receive any vaccinations whilst on chloramphenicol treatment.

Ciprofloxacin

Class: Quinolone antibiotic

Indications
- Mainly Gram-negative infections (e.g. *Salmonella* spp., *Pseudomonas* spp., *Campylobacter* spp., *Neisseria* spp., *Escherichia coli*, *Haemophilus influenzae*)
- Some Gram-positive infections (e.g. *Streptococcus pneumoniae*, *Enterococcus faecalis*)

Mechanism of action
- Ciprofloxacin is a broad-spectrum bactericidal antibiotic.
- It inhibits the activity of the bacterial enzyme DNA gyrase, which is necessary for coiling and replication of bacterial DNA. Human cells do not contain DNA gyrase.

Adverse effects
- *Common*: nausea, vomiting, abdominal pain, diarrhoea
- *Rare*: insomnia, confusion, convulsions, hepatitis, tendon damage, photosensitivity

Contraindications
- None
- Caution:
  - Epilepsy (ciprofloxacin lowers the seizure threshold)
  - Pregnancy
  - Breastfeeding
  - Children (animal studies have shown damage to cartilage)

Interactions
- *Ciclosporin*: concomitant use of ciprofloxacin and ciclosporin increases the risk of nephrotoxicity
- *Theophylline*: ciprofloxacin may increase the risk of convulsions
- *Warfarin*: ciprofloxacin enhances the anticoagulant effect of warfarin

Route of administration
- Oral, IV, eye drops

Note
- Clinically ciprofloxacin is used in respiratory tract, GI tract and complicated urinary tract infections. It is also used in gonorrhoea and in anthrax infections.
- Ciprofloxacin is mainly used to treat bacterial infections that are resistant to other commonly used antibiotics. Bacteria may become resistant to quinolones due to a mutation in their DNA gyrase. There is now a high incidence of resistant staphylococci.

Related drugs
- Cinoxacin, grepafloxacin, levofloxacin, nalidixic acid, norfloxacin, ofloxacin

Clotrimazole

Class: Imidazole antifungal

Indications
- Superficial, vaginal and mucous membrane fungal infections

Mechanism of action
- Clotrimazole is a broad-spectrum antifungal agent.
- It inhibits production of ergosterol (a steroid) in the fungal cell wall. This renders the cell wall unstable with ensuing efflux of phosphorus compounds, which in turn leads to breakdown of nucleic acids in the cell and potassium efflux. These actions result in fungal cell death.

Adverse effects
- *Rare*: dyspareunia (with vaginal application), GI upset, itching, rash, reversible liver damage

Contraindications
- First trimester of pregnancy

Interactions
- *Tacrolimus:* concomitant use may result in an increased plasma concentration of tacrolimus

Route of administration
- Topical, vaginal, oral

Note
- Clinically clotrimazole is used in dermatophyte, yeast and *Malassezia furfur* infections.
- Triazole antifunglas such as itraconazole are more specific towards fungal enzymes than imidazoles. This results in fewer adverse effects.
- Clotrimazole should not be applied in proximity of the eyes.

Related drugs
- Econazole, isoconazole, ketoconazole, miconazole, tioconazole

Erythromycin

Class: Macrolide antibiotic

Indications
- Alternative to penicillin in penicillin allergy
- Infections caused by Gram-positive (e.g. *Corynebacterium diphtheriae*) and some Gram-negative bacteria (e.g. *Bordetella pertussis*)
- *Mycoplasma pneumoniae*, *Legionella pneumophila*, *Treponema pallidum* and *Chlamydia* spp. infections
- Acne
- Rosacea

Mechanism of action
- Erythromycin is a broad-spectrum bacteriostatic antibiotic.
- It inhibits bacterial protein synthesis by reversibly binding to the 50S subunit of the bacterial ribosome.

Adverse effects
- *Common*: nausea, vomiting, abdominal pain, rash, phlebitis (when injected into a peripheral vein)
- *Rare*: reversible hearing loss (with high doses); cholestatic jaundice (with therapy lasting longer than 2 weeks), pseudomembranous colitis

Contraindications
- None
- Caution:
  - Liver disease
  - Renal impairment
  - Pregnancy
  - Breastfeeding

Interactions
- *Ciclosporin*: erythromycin increases the plasma concentration of ciclosporin
- *Digoxin*: the effects of digoxin are enhanced by erythromycin
- *Theophylline*: erythromycin increases the plasma concentration of theophylline
- *Warfarin*: erythromycin enhances the anticoagulant effect of warfarin
- *Note*: Erythromycin inhibits hepatic drug-metabolising enzymes; hence a wide range of further interactions exists

Route of administration
- Oral, IV

Note
- A course of erythromycin of longer than 14 days increases the risk of hepatic damage.

Related drugs
- Azithromycin, clarithromycin, roxithromicin, spiramicin

Flucloxacillin

Class: Beta-lactam antibiotic

Indications
- Beta-lactam-resistant *Staphylococcus* spp. infections (e.g. otitis externa, cellulitis)

Mechanism of action
- Flucloxacillin is a narrow-spectrum bactericidal antibiotic.
- It inhibits bacterial cell wall synthesis by preventing cross-linking between peptidoglycan chains that constitute the bacterial cell wall.

Adverse effects
- *Common*: hypersensitivity (rash, urticaria, fever, joint pains)
- *Rare*: anaphylaxis, cholestatic jaundice, hepatitis

Contraindications
- Penicillin hypersensitivity

Interactions
- *COC pill*: flucloxacillin can reduce the contraceptive effect by interfering with gut flora

Route of administration
- Oral, IM, IV

Note
- Unlike other penicillins, flucloxacillin is resistant to staphylococcal beta-lactamase. This bacterial enzyme cleaves the beta-lactam ring of other penicillins by hydrolysis, rendering them inactive.
- Flucloxacillin-resistant strains of *Staphylococcus aureus* (i.e. MRSA) have emerged in many hospitals. Therapy with vancomicin or teicoplanin is usually indicated for these organisms.
- Patients taking both the COC pill and flucloxacillin must be informed of the reduced contraceptive effect.
- The risk of cholestatic jaundice is increased if flucloxacillin is given for longer than 2 weeks.

Related drugs
- Cloxacillin, dicloxacillin

Gentamicin

Class: Aminoglycoside antibiotic

Indications
- Serious infections caused by aerobic Gram-negative bacteria
- Staphylococcal infections

Mechanism of action
- Gentamicin is bactericidal.
- Gentamicin inhibits bacterial protein synthesis by binding irreversibly to the 30S subunit of the bacterial ribosome.

Adverse effects
- *Rare*: nephrotoxicity, ototoxicity (gentamicin can damage the 8th cranial nerve), hypersensitivity reaction, grey baby syndrome in neonates

Contraindications
- Myasthenia gravis
- Caution:
  - Pregnancy (gentamicin crosses the placenta and can damage the fetal 8th cranial nerve)
  - Renal impairment

Interactions
- *Ciclosporin*: this potentiates nephrotoxic effects of gentamicin
- *Cytotoxics*: these potentiate nephrotoxic effects of gentamicin
- *Loop diuretics*: these potentiate ototoxic effects of gentamicin
- *Neostigmine, pyridostigmine*: gentamicin antagonises the effects of these drugs

Route of administration
- IV, IM, topical (eye drops), intrathecal

Note
- Gentamicin is not usually given for longer than 10 consecutive days because of potential ototoxicity and nephrotoxicity.
- It has a narrow therapeutic window, therefore therapeutic drug monitoring is essential (peak and trough concentrations are monitored).
- Gentamicin is usually combined with penicillin and/or metronidazole in blind therapy for serious infections.
- Amikacin can be used to treat serious infections caused by Gram-negative bacilli that are resistant to gentamicin.
- Gentamicin can cause grey baby syndrome in neonates. The grey skin discoloration is a consequence of tissue hypoperfusion and shock.

Related drugs
- Amikacin, kanamycin, neomycin, netilmicin, streptomycin, tobramycin

Metronidazole

Class: Nitroimidazole antibiotic

Indications
- Anaerobic and protozoal infections
- Part of *Helicobacter pylori* eradication therapy
- Rosacea
- Pseudomembranous colitis

Mechanism of action
- Metronidazole is a bacteriostatic antibiotic.
- It is broken down into toxic compounds (free radicals) within microbes that possess anaerobic or microaerophilic metabolism. These toxic compounds arrest growth by interfering with their nucleic acid function and synthesis.

Adverse effects
- *Common*: nausea, vomiting, anorexia, diarrhoea
- *Rare*: anaphylaxis, drowsiness, headache, dizziness, metallic taste in the mouth, peripheral neuropathy with long-term use

Contraindications
- None
- Caution:
  - Pregnancy and breastfeeding
  - Hepatic impairment

Interactions
- *Alcohol*: this causes a disulfiram-like reaction with metronidazole (see below)
- *Phenytoin*: metronidazole increases the plasma concentration of phenytoin by inhibiting its metabolism
- *Warfarin*: metronidazole enhances the anticoagulant effect of warfarin by inhibiting its metabolism

Route of administration
- Oral, IV, rectal

Note
- Therapeutic drug monitoring is advised for treatment exceeding 10 days.
- Metronidazole is commonly used to treat dental infections as these are mostly caused by anaerobes. It is also widely used as prophylaxis and treatment of intra-abdominal infections.
- Patients should be warned of the disulfiram-like reaction that occurs if alcohol is taken while on metronidazole treatment (flushing, abdominal pain, hypotension). This reaction can occur up to 3 days after stopping treatment.

Related drugs
- Ornidazole, tinidazole

Rifampicin

Class: Antituberculous agent

Indications
- Tuberculosis
- Leprosy
- Prophylaxis of meningococcal meningitis and *Haemophilus influenzae* type b infection in contacts of cases

Mechanism of action
- Rifampicin inhibits the DNA-dependent RNA polymerase isoenzyme in bacteria (but not in human cells) and is thus bactericidal.

Adverse effects
- *Common*: disturbance of LFTs; orange-coloured tears, urine and sputum
- *Rare*: hepatitis, rash, thrombocytopenia, nausea, vomiting, flu-like illness, orange discoloration of soft contact lenses

Contraindications
- Jaundice

Interactions
- *Calcium channel blockers, corticosteroids and phenytoin*: rifampicin accelerates the metabolism of these drugs, thus reducing their effects
- *Oestrogens and progestogens*: rifampicin accelerates the metabolism of the COC pill, thus reducing the contraceptive effect
- *Warfarin*: rifampicin increases the metabolism of warfarin, thus decreasing its effect
- *Note*: Rifampicin induces hepatic drug-metabolising enzymes; hence a wide range of further interactions exists

Route of administration
- Oral, IV

Note
- Resistance to rifampicin can develop rapidly if it is used alone. Therefore it is usually given in combination with ethambutol, pyrazinamide and isoniazid in patients with tuberculosis.
- LFTs should be carried out before treatment. The patient should be advised how to recognise signs of liver dysfunction. If these occur, LFTs should be repeated.
- Compliance may be difficult, as treatment for tuberculosis lasts for 6–9 months.

Tetracycline

Class: Tetracycline antibiotic

Indications
- Infections caused by *Coxiella burnetii*, *Mycoplasma* spp., *Leptospira ictohaemorrhagiae*, *Chlamydia* spp., *Rickettsia* spp., *Borrellia burgdorferi* and other susceptible organisms
- Acne
- Rosacea

Mechanism of action
- Tetracycline is a broad-spectrum bacteriostatic antibiotic.
- It undergoes selective uptake into bacterial cells and binds reversibly to the 30S subunit of the ribosome. This disrupts protein synthesis by interfering with RNA translation.

Adverse effects
- *Common*: nausea, vomiting, diarrhoea
- *Rare*: acute renal failure, photosensitivity, pruritus ani, black hairy tongue, pancreatitis

Contraindications
- Children
- Pregnancy
- Breastfeeding
- Renal impairment
- SLE

Interactions
- *Antacids*: these decrease the absorption of tetracycline
- *Ferrous sulphate*: tetracycline decreases the absorption of ferrous sulphate

Route of administration
- Oral, topical, IM, IV

Note
- Most Gram-positive and several Gram-negative bacteria are now resistant to tetracycline (resistance is mediated by plasmids).
- Tetracycline binds to calcium and is therefore deposited in growing bones and teeth. This leads to discoloration of teeth and should therefore not be given to children under 12 years of age or to lactating or pregnant women.
- Tetracycline should not be taken with food or milk (impaired absorption).
- Doxycycline is preferred to tetracycline as it does not affect renal function and its absorption is not decreased by milk.

Related drugs
- Doxycycline, lymecycline, minocycline, oxytetracycline

Trimethoprim

Class: Antifolate antibiotic

Indications
- Treatment and prophylaxis of UTIs
- Prostatitis

Mechanism of action
- Trimethoprim reduces bacterial production of folate by inhibiting the bacterial enzyme dihydrofolate reductase. Trimethoprim has a 50 000 times greater affinity for bacterial dihydrofolate reductase than for human dihydrofolate reductase.
- Trimethoprim is bacteriostatic, as folate is an essential cofactor in DNA synthesis.

Adverse effects
- *Rare*: bone marrow suppression, nausea, vomiting, rash, toxic epidermal necrolysis

Contraindications
- Pregnancy (due to teratogenic risk)
- Blood disorders (e.g. anaemia, thrombocytopenia)

Interactions
- *Ciclosporin*: concomitant use of ciclosporin and trimethoprim increases the risk of nephrotoxicity
- *Cytotoxics*: concomitant use increases the risk of bone marrow toxicity
- *Pyrimethamine*: concomitant use of pyrimethamine and trimethoprim can enhance the antifolate effect

Route of administration
- Oral, IV

Note
- Resistance to trimethoprim is common.
- Folate deficiency can be avoided by giving folinic acid.
- Trimethoprim can be used in combination with sulphamethoxazole (a sulphonamide) as co-trimoxazole, which is bactericidal. This combination produces synergistic activity and is especially effective for *Pneumocystis carinii* infections.

Vancomicin

Class: Glycopeptide antibiotic

Indications
- Infections caused by Gram-positive cocci, in particular MRSA
- Pseudomembranous colitis (caused by *Clostridium difficile*)

Mechanism of action
- Vancomicin is a bactericidal antibiotic.
- It inhibits bacterial cell wall synthesis by binding to precursor units of the cell wall.
- Vancomicin also interferes with RNA synthesis and permeability of the bacterial cell wall.

Adverse effects
- *Common*: anorexia, nausea
- *Rare*: agranulocytosis, 'red man' syndrome (flushing of the upper body), rash, renal failure, hearing loss, GI upset, fever, chills

Contraindications
- Hypersensitivity

Interactions
- *Ciclosporin*: the risk of nephrotoxicity is increased
- *Loop diuretics*: the risk of ototoxicity is increased
- *Oestrogens*: possible reduced contraceptive effect

Route of administration
- Oral (for pseudomembranous or other colitis), IV

Note
- Clinically vancomicin is used in staphylococcal enterocolitis or other staphylococcal infections (e.g. endocarditis).
- Agranulocytosis can occur one or more weeks after starting IV vancomicin. It is often reversible by stopping vancomicin.
- Vancomicin resistant enterococci (VRE) strains first emerged in 1987 and have spread rapidly since then. Prevention of VRE relies on good hygiene (e.g. hand washing) and careful, restricted use of vancomicin.

Related drugs
- Teicoplanin

Zidovudine

Class: Nucleoside reverse transcriptase inhibitor (NRTI)

Indications
- Part of combination therapy for HIV infection
- Prevention of HIV transmission from mother to fetus

Mechanism of action
- Zidovudine is a nucleoside analogue. It is phosphorylated inside cells to form zidovudine triphosphate, which is a competitive inhibitor of viral reverse transcriptase. Zidovudine triphosphate is also incorporated into proviral DNA, thus terminating DNA chain elongation.
- NB: zidovudine does not eradicate HIV from the body.

Adverse effects
- *Common*: anaemia, neutropenia, headache, insomnia, nausea, abdominal pain
- *Rare*: convulsions, myalgia, myopathy

Contraindications
- Low neutrophil count
- Severe anaemia
- Breastfeeding

Interactions
- *Ganciclovir*: severe myelosuppression if given with zidovudine
- *Probenecid*: this increases the risk of zidovudine toxicity by raising its plasma concentration

Route of administration
- Oral, IV

Note
- Resistance to zidovudine develops as a result of mutations in viral reverse transcriptase. Combined therapy is given in order to prevent emergence of resistant strains (see p. 132)
- Therapy is guided by HIV viral load and CD4 count.
- Blood transfusions are frequently required as zidovudine commonly causes anaemia.

Related drugs
- Abacavir, didanosine, lamivudine, stavudine, tenofovir disoproxil, zalcitabine

IMMUNISATION

RECOMMENDED IMMUNISATION PROGRAMME IN THE UK

Vaccine	Age
Hepatitis B (for infants at risk)	Birth, 1 month and 6 months
DTP, poliomyelitis, Hib, Meningococcal Group C	2, 3 and 4 months
MMR	12 months
DT, poliomyelitis, MMR	3–5 years (pre-school booster)
BCG	10–14 years (given at birth if at risk)
DT (low dose), poliomyelitis	13–18 years (school-leavers)

Note
· If the immunisation course is interrupted, there is no need to
restart the entire course.
· Jet guns should not be used for vaccination due to the risk of
transmission of blood-borne infections.
· Immunisation schedules may differ between countries.
National immunisation guidelines should be consulted.

CONTRAINDICATIONS TO ALL VACCINES
· Acute febrile illness
· Severe reaction to a previous dose

CONTRAINDICATIONS TO LIVE VACCINES
(BCG, MMR, POLIOMYELITIS)
· Acute febrile illness
· Severe reaction to a previous dose
· Immunocompromised patients
· Pregnancy

- HIV (omit BCG, but MMR and inactivated poliomyelitis vaccine can be given)
- High-dose corticosteroids (wait for 3 months after stopping steroids)
- Chemo/radiotherapy (wait for 6 months after stopping therapy)
- Another live vaccine within the previous 3 weeks
- Certain malignant conditions (e.g. leukaemia, malignancy of the reticuloendothelial system)

BCG vaccine (Bacillus Calmette–Guérin)

Class: Live attenuated vaccine

Indications
- Prophylaxis of tuberculosis
- Primary or recurrent carcinoma of the bladder

Mechanism of action
- BCG vaccine contains a live attenuated strain derived from *Mycobacterium bovis*. This induces a hypersensitivity reaction and thereby stimulates cell-mediated immunity against *Mycobacterium tuberculosis*.
- Instillation into the bladder results in chronic granulomatous cystitis, an immunological response thought to be essential for antitumour activity.

Adverse effects
- *Common*: ulcer at injection site
- *Rare*: axillary lymphadenopathy, tuberculosis (in the immunocompromised); cystitis, haematuria, urinary frequency, systemic BCG infection (with bladder instillation)

Contraindications
- Acute febrile illness
- Immunocompromised patients (e.g. steroid therapy, immunosuppressive drugs, HIV, malignancy)
- Pregnancy
- Chemo/radiotherapy (defer BCG vaccine for 6 months)
- The first 3 weeks following another live vaccine
- Malignant conditions of the reticuloendothelial system
- Leukaemia

Interactions
- None

Route of administration
- Intradermal, topical

Note
- BCG vaccine should only be given if the Heaf test or Mantoux test is negative (with exception of infants < 3 months of age).
- An ulcer usually appears at the site of injection 2–3 weeks after the vaccination. This normally heals within 6–12 weeks.
- It is standard practice to give the vaccine into the left upper arm so that BCG status can be easily checked. The injection leaves a characteristic scar for life.
- Traumatic catheterisation during bladder instillation of BCG may lead to systemic BCG infection. This usually responds well to antituberculous drugs.

Diphtheria vaccine

Class: Toxoid vaccine

Indications
- Prophylaxis of diphtheria

Mechanism of action
- Diphtheria vaccine contains inactivated diphtheria toxin (toxoid), which stimulates production of antibodies. These provide immunity against *Corynebacterium diphtheriae*.

Adverse effects
- *Common*: pain and swelling at the site of injection
- *Rare*: fever, arthralgia

Contraindications
- Acute febrile illness
- Severe reaction to a previous dose

Interactions
- None

Route of administration
- IM, deep subcutaneous

Note
- The vaccine is given to children as part of the triple vaccine (DTP vaccine). It is also given to travellers going to areas where diphtheria is prevalent.
- Adults and children over 10 years of age who require a primary dose or a booster should be given the low-dose vaccine.

Hepatitis B vaccine

Class: Subunit vaccine

Indications
- Prophylaxis of hepatitis B

Mechanism of action
- The vaccine contains HBsAg, which is prepared in yeast by recombinant DNA technology. It stimulates production of anti-HBsAg antibodies, which confer protective immunity.

Adverse effects
- *Common*: discomfort at the injection site
- *Rare*: anaphylaxis, thrombocytopenia

Contraindications
- Acute febrile illness
- Severe reaction to a previous dose

Interactions
- None

Route of administration
- IM (deltoid muscle, not gluteal), subcutaneous (to avoid bleeding in haemophilia patients)

Note
- Hepatitis B vaccine should be given to those at high risk (e.g. health care workers, haemophiliacs, babies born to infected mothers).
- The vaccine takes up to 6 months to achieve a protective level of antibodies. Boosters every 5 years are recommended.
- Following a single episode of exposure to hepatitis B virus (e.g. contact with infected blood), injection of hepatitis B–specific immunoglobulin should be given as soon as possible. This confers a significant level of protection against the disease.

Hib vaccine (*Haemophilus influenzae* type b)

Class: Inactivated vaccine

Indications
- Prophylaxis of Hib infections

Mechanism of action
- Hib vaccine contains a capsular polysaccharide obtained from *Haemophilus influenzae* type b, which has been conjugated to a protein carrier (this enhances immunogenicity). Administration stimulates an antibody response.

Adverse effects
- *Common*: local erythema, fever, headache, anorexia, diarrhoea, vomiting
- *Rare*: convulsions, erythema multiforme, anaphylaxis

Contraindications
- Acute febrile illness
- Severe reaction to a previous dose
- Pregnancy
- Breastfeeding

Interactions
- None

Route of administration
- IM, deep subcutaneous

Note
- The goal of vaccination is to prevent Hib epiglottitis and meningitis.
- Hib vaccine is not usually required for children over 4 years of age because the risk of infection with Hib falls rapidly after this age. Exceptions to this rule are patients with sickle-cell disease, asplenic patients and those on treatment for malignancy.
- As Hib vaccine contains traces of cow's brain tissue, there is potentially a minimal risk of transmission of Creutzfeldt–Jacob disease.

Meningococcal Group C vaccine

Class: Conjugate or polysaccharide vaccine

Indications
- Prophylaxis of *Neisseria meningitidis* serogroup C meningitis

Mechanism of action
- The vaccine contains group C–specific meningococcal polysaccharides, which stimulate the immune system to produce protective antibodies.

Adverse effects
- *Common*: erythema and swelling at the site of injection, fever, headache
- *Rare*: seizures, hypersensitivity, meningism

Contraindications
- Acute febrile illness
- Severe reaction to a previous dose

Interactions
- None

Route of administration
- IM, subcutaneous

Note
- 40% of cases of meningitis are caused by group C *Neisseria meningitidis*, the remaining 60% being caused by group B strain.
- There are 2 types of meningococcal C vaccine in use:
  1 Group C conjugate vaccine: a conjugate between a protein carrier and group C–specific capsular polysaccharide
  2 Polysaccharide vaccine: a combination of group C–specific polysaccharides
- Meningococcal vaccine should be given to patients up to the age of 24 who have not been previously immunised. As the risk of meningitis declines with age, immunisation is not usually indicated in those over 25 years of age.
- Meningococcal vaccine should also be given to those with an absent or dysfunctional spleen (conjugate vaccine).
- Travellers to high-risk countries (e.g. Africa, Saudi Arabia) should be offered the meningococcal polysaccharide vaccine.

MMR vaccine (measles, mumps, rubella)

Class: Combined live-attenuated vaccine

Indications
- Prophylaxis of measles, mumps and rubella

Mechanism of action
- MMR vaccine contains live-attenuated strains of measles, mumps and rubella viruses.
- It provides active immunity by stimulating an antibody-mediated response.

Adverse effects
- *Common*: fever, malaise, rash
- *Rare*: parotid swelling, idiopathic thrombocytopenic purpura

Contraindications
- Immunocompromised children
- Pregnancy
- Another live vaccine within the previous 3 weeks
- Allergy to neomycin or kanamycin (MMR vaccine contains traces of both)
- Acute febrile illness
- Severe reaction to a previous dose
- Chemo/radiotherapy (defer the vaccine for 6 weeks)
- Leukaemia
- Malignant conditions of the reticuloendothelial system

Interactions
- None

Route of administration
- IM, deep subcutaneous

Note
- Women should avoid pregnancy for 1 month following MMR vaccination.
- MMR vaccine does not provide effective protection following exposure to mumps or rubella virus because the antibody response to these components of the vaccine is too slow.
- Adverse effects commonly occur following the first dose and much less so following the second dose of MMR vaccine.
- The link between MMR vaccine and both autism and inflammatory bowel disease has been disproved.
- MMR vaccine should be administered irrespective of previous infection with mumps, measles or rubella.

Pertussis vaccine

Class: Inactivated vaccine

Indications
- Prophylaxis of whooping cough

Mechanism of action
- Pertussis vaccine contains killed *Bordetella pertussis* organisms. The vaccine induces active immunity by formation of antibodies against *Bordetella pertussis*.

Adverse effects
- *Common*: fever, pain and redness at the site of injection
- *Rare*: encephalopathy, convulsions, oedema and induration of the limb into which the injection was given

Contraindications
- Acute febrile illness
- Severe reaction to a previous dose

Interactions
- None

Route of administration
- IM, deep subcutaneous

Note
- Acellular pertussis vaccine is given to those who have had a serious reaction to a previous dose. It is only available on a named patient basis.

Poliomyelitis vaccine

Class: Live-attenuated or inactivated vaccine

Indications
- Prophylaxis of poliomyelitis

Mechanism of action
- The oral poliomyelitis vaccine (Sabin vaccine) contains live-attenuated strains of polioviruses. It induces active immunity by formation of IgG and IgA antibodies, thereby conferring protection against poliomyelitis infections of the CNS and GI tract.
- The inactivated subcutaneous vaccine (Salk vaccine) induces the formation of IgG antibodies and to a lesser extent IgA antibodies. It induces only little immunity in the intestinal tract but confers protection against polio infections of the CNS.

Adverse effects
- *Rare*: paralysis with oral vaccine (less than 1 in 2 million doses)

Contraindications
- Sabin vaccine (oral):
  - Vomiting and diarrhoea
  - Immunosuppression
  - Pregnancy
  - Severe reaction to a previous dose
  - Malignancy
  - Chemo/radiotherapy (defer the vaccine for 6 months)

Interactions
- None

Route of administration
- Salk vaccine: subcutaneous
- Sabin vaccine: oral

Note
- Salk vaccine is used only if Sabin vaccine is contraindicated due to immunosuppression.
- Poliomyelitis is endemic in developing countries and therefore non-immunised travellers to countries other than New Zealand, Australia, North America or Northern or Western Europe should be vaccinated (unless previously vaccinated).
- Orally vaccinated children are usually infectious to others for about 6 weeks due to shedding of the virus in the faeces.

Tetanus vaccine

Class: Toxoid vaccine

Indications
- Prophylaxis of tetanus

Mechanism of action
- Tetanus vaccine contains inactivated tetanus toxin (toxoid), which stimulates antibody-mediated active immunity.

Adverse effects
- *Common*: pain and tenderness at the site of injection
- *Rare*: fever

Contraindications
- Acute febrile illness
- Severe reaction to a previous dose

Interactions
- None

Route of administration
- IM

Note
- A full course of tetanus immunisation should be given to both non-immunised individuals and to those with unknown immunisation status following a penetrating injury or burns (three vaccines given monthly and a booster every 10 years).
- Following an injury in a previously immunised individual, a booster should be given only if more than 10 years have elapsed since the last administration.

Management guidelines (pp. 165–168)
Contraception
Hormone replacement therapy
Hypertension in pregnancy
Induction of labour
Menorrhagia
Polycystic ovary syndrome
Pre-eclampsia
    Eclampsia

Individual drugs (pp. 168–172)
Ergometrine; Oestrogens; Oxytocin; Progestogens; Tranexamic acid

CONTRACEPTION
• 90% of fertile young females who have regular unprotected intercourse become pregnant within 1 year

Methods of contraception
1 Natural methods: rhythm method, coitus interruptus
2 Barrier methods: male or female condom, diaphragm, cervical cap
3 IUCD: These are unsuitable contraception for women with heavy or painful periods. IUCDs usually last a minimum of 5 years.
4 Mirena device: a progesterone-loaded IUCD, especially useful for women with heavy periods
5 Hormonal: COC pill, POP, subcutaneous medroxyprogesterone depot injection (usually lasts 8–12 weeks), subcutaneous implant (usually lasts 3–5 years)
6 Sterilisation: vasectomy in males (failure rate of about 1 in 2000), laparoscopic occlusion of the fallopian tubes in females (failure rate of about 1 in 200)

Risks and benefits of the COC pill
• Giving oestrogens alone involves a risk of developing breast cancer or endometrial cancer in women with a uterus. For this reason oestrogen is combined with a progestogen in the COC pill.
• Oestrogen can also predispose to thromboembolic events. Women who are obese, diabetic, smoke or have any other additional risk factors for thromboembolic events should either be warned about the risks or should be declined the COC pill, if appropriate.
• The COC pill furthermore protects against pelvic infection/PID, ovarian cancer, ovarian cysts and benign breast disease.

Progestogen-only pill ('Mini-pill')
• The POP is given when COCs are contraindicated (e.g. history of thromboembolic disease). However, the POP has a slightly higher failure rate than the COC pill.
• The POP must be taken at the same time each day. The contraceptive effect is inadequate if administration is delayed by more than 3 h. In this case the pill should be continued as normal, but a different method of contraception (e.g. condom) should be used for a period of 1 week.

Post-coital contraception
• 'Morning-after pill' (contains levonorgestrel) – give one dose within 72 h following unprotected sexual intercourse, followed by a second dose 12 h later
• Alternatively, an IUCD can be placed within 5 days following unprotected intercourse

HORMONE REPLACEMENT THERAPY
• **Climacteric**: this is the time of waning fertility leading up to the menopause
• **Menopause**: the time of the last menstrual cycle; average age in the UK is 51
• **Premature menopause**: this occurs in about 1% of women in the UK, and is defined as the last menstrual cycle occurring before the age of 40
• HRT consists of regular oestrogen and progesterone given for a period of up to 5 years once the menopause has been reached. It can be given orally or as a patch, gel or subcutaneous implant. HRT aims to counter the changes brought on by the menopause, which are due to a lack of oestrogens. It should not be given for any other reason than to relieve postmenopausal symptoms.
• Women on HRT need to be reviewed yearly to assess the need for ongoing HRT.

Benefits of HRT
1 Symptomatic relief of postmenopausal symptoms (e.g. flushing, sweating, mood changes, thinning hair, wrinkling skin)
2 Prevention of menopause-associated disease processes (e.g. osteoporosis, ovarian cancer)
3 A progestogen is added to HRT in order to prevent cystic hyperplasia and oestrogen-related cancer of the endometrium

Disadvantages of HRT
1 Adverse effects of oestrogen and progestogen
2 Increased risk of breast cancer
3 Recent evidence suggests an increased risk of CHD and dementia

Contraindications to HRT
• Pregnancy and breastfeeding
• Oestrogen-dependent cancer (such as endometrial and breast cancer)
• Thromboembolic disorders
• Liver disease
• Undiagnosed vaginal bleeding

HYPERTENSION IN PREGNANCY
• Admit if BP exceeds 160/100 mmHg in a known hypertensive
• Advise bed rest
• Monitor BP 2–4-hourly, urine protein by urinalysis, plasma urate and LFTs, platelet count and the fetus (CTG)
• If high BP persists, treat with antihypertensives (see below)
• If high BP persists with proteinuria, treat as for pre-eclampsia

Pharmacological treatment
• Treat if BP reaches 160/105 mmHg
• Drugs that are commonly used:
  1 Oral methyldopa
  2 Oral beta blocker (e.g. labetolol)
  3 Oral nifedipine

INDUCTION OF LABOUR
• Assess the state of the cervix prior to induction using the Bishop score (this assesses station, position and cervical effacement/consistency/dilatation)
• Unripe cervix must be ripened with vaginal prostaglandins (e.g. PGE$_2$)
• If this fails, consider Caesarean section
• Once the cervix is ripe, rupture the membranes
• Monitor fetal heart with CTG
• If necessary, give IV oxytocin until effective uterine contractions are present (sometimes given until delivery)
• A combination of IM ergometrine and oxytocin is given to the mother when the baby's anterior shoulder is delivered. This accelerates the 3rd stage of labour and reduces the risk of postpartum haemorrhage
• NB: an induction should always be managed as high-risk labour

MENORRHAGIA
• Treat any underlying cause (e.g. pelvic pathology, clotting disorder, medical disorders)
• In most cases no organic cause is found (termed dysfunctional uterine bleeding) and treatment is mainly symptomatic:
  1 Medical treatment

- To decrease blood loss: antifibrinolytics (e.g. tranexamic acid), NSAIDs (e.g. mefenamic acid) or systemic progestogens
- To restore a regular cycle: COC pill
2 Progesterone-loaded IUCD (Mirena)
3 Surgical treatment
  - Endometrial resection or ablation
  - Myomectomy for fibroids (only performed if further pregnancies are desired or patient is unwilling to have hysterectomy, as the complication rate of myomectomy is greater than that of hysterectomy)
  - Hysterectomy in severe cases

POLYCYSTIC OVARY SYNDROME
- Incidence is about 20–30% of women, but only 10% are symptomatic and therefore may need treatment
- Encourage weight loss, if appropriate
- For regulation of menstruation: COC pill
- For hirsutism/acne:
  - COC pill containing cyproterone acetate
  - Alternatively, hirsutism may be treated by depilation (waxing), electrolysis or laser hair removal
- If pregnancy is desired:
  - Clomiphene (an oestrogen antagonist acting on the hypothalamus) – this induces ovulation in about 70% of women given clomiphene
  - If clomiphene fails, consider gonadotrophins
- NB: it is important to monitor serum or urine oestrogen levels to detect any developing ovarian hyperstimulation

PRE-ECLAMPSIA
- The objective of treatment is to prevent eclampsia
- Admit if BP is > 140/90 mmHg with proteinuria and oedema
- Monitor BP 2–4-hourly, 24-h urine protein, plasma urate, platelets and LFTs (especially ALT, AST), and the fetus (CTG)
- If BP is > 150/105 mmHg, control with antihypertensives to prevent maternal intracranial haemorrhage: IV hydralazine or IV labetalol or oral nifedipine
- Advise bed rest
- The mother must be monitored after delivery, as eclampsia can occur post partum (especially within the first 48 h)
- Beware of warning signs of eclampsia: epigastric pain, headaches, blurred vision

ECLAMPSIA (maternal convulsions during pregnancy)
- Lie the patient on her left side
- Give oxygen
- Give IV magnesium sulphate to control fits

- Give IV hydralazine or IV labetalol to control BP
- Once BP and fits are controlled, deliver the baby
- Check magnesium levels, test patellar reflexes regularly and monitor urine output after giving magnesium sulphate (loss of reflexes is an early sign of toxicity; magnesium sulphate is excreted in the urine)
- The mother must be monitored after delivery, as eclampsia can occur post partum (especially within the first 48 h)
- NB: delivery is the only cure

Ergometrine

Class: Ergot alkaloid

Indications
- Prevention and treatment of postpartum haemorrhage
- Active management of the 3rd stage of labour
- Uterine bleeding due to an incomplete abortion

Mechanism of action
- Exact mechanism is not fully understood.
- It may act at alpha adrenoceptors, prostaglandin and serotonin receptors in smooth muscle.
- Ergometrine causes uterine contractions and has some degree of vasoconstrictor action.

Adverse effects
- *Common*: nausea, vomiting, abdominal pain, hypertension, headache, dizziness
- *Rare*: palpitations, tingling in fingers, anginal pain

Contraindications
- Induction of labour
- 1st and 2nd stages of labour
- Eclampsia
- Hypertension
- Peripheral vascular disease and CHD (due to vasoconstrictor action)
- Severe cardiac, hepatic or renal impairment
- Sepsis

Interactions
- *Macrolide antibiotics*: increased risk of ergotism (nausea, vomiting, visual disturbances, peripheral ischaemia)
- *Protease inhibitors*: increased risk of ergotism
- *Tetracycline*: increased risk of ergotism

Route of administration
- Oral, IM, IV (in emergencies)

Note
- IM ergometrine is often given together with oxytocin in the 3rd stage of labour or in postpartum haemorrhage. These two drugs, when combined, are more effective than either one of them alone.
- Due to its vasoconstrictor action, ergometrine may cause spasm of the coronary arteries, resulting in anginal pain.
- Ergometrine will cause an inappropriately relaxed uterus to contract, aiming to reduce bleeding from the placental bed. It exerts little effect on an already contracted uterus.

Oestrogens

Class: Sex hormones

Indications
- Contraception (in the form of the COC pill)
- Hormone replacement therapy
- Atrophic vaginitis (topical use only)

Mechanism of action
- In HRT, replacing the deficient oestrogen alleviates menopausal symptoms.
- Given as the COC pill, oestrogens inhibit the release of FSH from the anterior pituitary by negative feedback. This prevents maturation of the Graafian follicle in the ovary.

Adverse effects
- *Common*: fluid retention, hypertension, loss of libido, nausea, vomiting, breast tenderness, weight gain, acne, mood swings, worsening of pre-existing migraine
- *Rare*: thromboembolic events, headache, depression, slightly increased risk of breast cancer, slightly increased risk of endometrial cancer (only if given alone without a progestogen), hepatic tumours, cholestatic jaundice

Contraindications
- Pregnancy
- Breastfeeding
- Previous thromboembolic events (e.g. PE)
- Active hepatic disease (oestrogens are metabolised by the liver)
- Oestrogen-dependent tumours (e.g. endometrial cancer)
- Focal migraine

Interactions
- *Broad-spectrum antibiotics*: these may decrease the effects of oestrogens by impairing the gut flora responsible for recycling ethinyloestradiol in the large bowel
- *Carbamazepine*: this increases the metabolism of oestrogens, thereby decreasing their effect
- *Phenytoin, rifampicin*: these drugs decrease the plasma concentration of oestrogens
- *Warfarin*: oestrogens reduce the anticoagulant effect of warfarin

Route of administration
- HRT: oral, transdermal patch, subcutaneous implant, gel
- Contraception: oral, subutaneous, IM
- Atrophic vaginitis: vaginal cream or pessary

Note
- Blood pressure should be checked regularly due to the risk of hypertension.
- The COC pill failure rate is 3–5 pregnancies per 100 woman-years of administration. This is largely due to incorrect self-administration.
- Oestrogens may need to be discontinued several weeks prior to surgery, as they predispose to thromboembolic events.

Oxytocin

Class: Oxytocic agent

Indications
- Induction or augmentation of labour
- Management of the 3rd stage of labour
- Prevention and treatment of postpartum haemorrhage
- Uterine bleeding after spontaneous or induced abortion

Mechanism of action
- Oxytocin produces contractions of the fundus in the pregnant uterus by acting on local oxytocin receptors.
- It also enhances uterine contractions by increasing the production of prostaglandins in the myometrium.

Adverse effects
- *Common*: uterine spasm, nausea, vomiting
- *Rare*: fluid and electrolyte disturbance, hypotension, tachycardia, cardiac dysrhythmias

Contraindications
- Mechanical obstruction in labour and any other condition where vaginal delivery is not advisable
- Predisposition to uterine rupture (e.g. previous Caesarean section)
- Fetal distress

Interactions
- *Sympathomimetics*: vasopressor effects are enhanced

Route of administration
- IV

Note
- Careful monitoring of fetal heart rate and uterine contractions is required when oxytocin is used in labour. This is due to the risk of fetal hypoxia caused by uterine hyperstimulation. Oxytocin should be discontinued in cases of uterine hyperactivity or fetal distress.
- Oxytocin is often given together with ergometrine in the 3rd stage of labour or in postpartum haemorrhage. These two drugs, when combined, are more effective than either one of them alone.
- Oxytocin is infused using IV fluids. If large amounts of oxytocin, and therefore fluids, are given, the patient may suffer hyponatraemic seizures secondary to water intoxication. This risk is increased by oxytocin's antidiuretic activity (it structurally resembles vasopressin).

Progestogens

Class: Sex hormones

Indications
- Contraception
- Part of hormone replacement therapy
- Menstrual disorders (e.g. dysmenorrhoea, menorrhagia)
- Endometriosis
- Neoplastic disease (endometrial cancer, renal cell carcinoma, 2nd or 3rd line therapy in the treatment of breast cancer)

Mechanism of action
- The main contraceptive effect of progestogens is due to their action on cervical mucus, which is rendered impenetrable to sperm. Progestogens also prevent implantation of the fertilised ovum by rendering the endometrium hostile.
- Progestogens immobilise sperm by increasing the pH of uterine fluid.
- Progestogens also suppress the secretion of gonadotrophins from the anterior pituitary by negative feedback, thus inhibiting ovulation in about 40% of females.
- In endometriosis, progestogens are used to inhibit menstruation, thus producing regression of small lesions.

Adverse effects
- *Common*: menstrual irregularities, breast tenderness, weight gain, acne, bloating, nausea, vomiting, hot flushes
- *Rare*: cholestatic jaundice, thromboembolism

Contraindications
- Pregnancy
- Severe hypertension
- Unexplained vaginal bleeding
- Hepatic impairment

Interactions
- *Rifamycins*: reduced contraceptive effect
- *Carbamazepine, phenytoin*: these drugs reduce the contraceptive effect
- *Ciclosporin*: progestogens increase the plasma concentration of ciclosporin
- *Warfarin*: reduced anticoagulant effect

Route of administration
- Oral, vaginal gel/pessary, rectal, IM, subdermal implant, IUCD

Note
- Progestogens are divided into two main classes:
  - progesterone with its analogues (hydroxyprogesterone, dydrogesterone, medroxyprogesterone)
  - testosterone with its analogues (norgestrel, norethisterone). Gestodene, desogestrel and norgestimate are derivatives of norgestrel.

Tranexamic acid

Class: Antifibrinolytic agent

Indications
- Menorrhagia
- Treatment and prevention of haemorrhage (e.g. haemophilia, perioperatively)
- Hereditary angioedema

Mechanism of action
- Tranexamic acid inhibits activation of plasminogen to plasmin, which is an essential factor in the fibrinolysis cascade. This action enhances clot stability.
- Tranexamic acid has no effect on platelets.

Adverse effects
- *Rare*: hypotension, thromboembolic events (including central retinal artery and vein obstruction), colour vision disturbance, dizziness, GI disturbance (diarrhoea, nausea, vomiting)

Contraindications
- Thromboembolic disorders
- Subarachnoid haemorrhage

Interactions
- None known

Route of administration
- Oral, IV

Note
- Tranexamic acid is used in dental, gynaecological and urological surgery in patients who have clotting disorders (e.g. von Willebrand's disease, haemophilia). It is not used in abdominal or thoracic surgery due to the risk of insoluble haematomas forming.
- Patients should be made aware of the symptoms of arterial or venous thrombembolism.

Related drugs
- Aminocaproic acid, aprotinin

ANAESTHESIA

General anaesthesia (pp. 173–174)
Premedication
Anaesthetic agents
Muscle-relaxing agents
Analgesic agents

Local anaesthesia (pp. 174–175)
Local IV regional anaesthesia (Bier's block)
Epidural anaesthesia
Spinal anaesthesia

Individual drugs (pp. 176–182)
Atracurium; Isoflurane; Lidocaine; Neostigmine; Nitrous oxide; Propofol

GENERAL ANAESTHESIA

General anaesthetic agents are employed as an adjunct to surgical procedures. They achieve a state of complete and reversible loss of consciousness in which the patient is unaware of and unresponsive to painful stimuli.

Unlike local anaesthetics, general anaesthetics are given systemically. They produce their effects by acting on the CNS, whilst maintaining the functioning of other body systems such as the cardiovascular and respiratory systems.

Agents used in general anaesthesia are manifold and can be divided into the following four categories:

1. Premedication (given before induction of general anaesthesia)
- Benzodiazepines to reduce anxiety
- Antimuscarinics (e.g. hyoscine, atropine) to reduce bronchial secretions and vagal reflexes
- Opioids for analgesic and sedative effects (give with an antiemetic)
- NB: the use of premedication is declining

2. Anaesthetic agents
- Induction of general anaesthesia by IV agents:
  - Non-barbiturates (e.g. propofol, ketamine, etomidate)
  - Barbiturates (e.g. thiopentone, methohexitone)
- Maintenance of anaesthesia by inhalational agents (e.g. isoflurane, sevoflurane, desflurane), but sometimes achieved with IV propofol alone (total IV anaesthesia)

3. Muscle-relaxing agents
- Depolarising (suxamethonium) and non-depolarising (e.g. atracurium) muscle relaxants are used to facilitate surgery and ventilation

- After surgery the effects of non-depolarising muscle relaxants are reversed by anticholinesterase drugs (neostigmine)
4. **Analgesic agents (**used perioperatively**)**
  - Paracetamol
  - NSAIDs (e.g. ibuprofen, diclofenac)
  - Opioids in conjunction with an antiemetic
  - Local anaesthetics (lidocaine, bupivacaine)

LOCAL ANAESTHESIA

Local anaesthesia is the method of choice for many minor surgical procedures. It is especially useful in patients suffering from severe cardiorespiratory disease who are more susceptible to the risks of general anaesthesia.

Agents used to induce local anaesthesia (e.g. lidocaine) act by causing a local nerve conduction block. The following types of local anaesthesia are used:
- Local infiltration
- Nerve block (e.g. ring block in a finger)
- Local IV regional anaesthesia (Bier's block)
- Central neural blockade (epidural/spinal anaesthesia)

Local IV regional anaesthesia (Bier's block)
- This technique provides good operating conditions for hand surgery or manual reduction of wrist/forearm fractures.
- A tourniquet is applied to the upper arm and inflated to 300 mmHg.
- Local anaesthetic (prilocaine) is then injected IV into the arm, distal to the tourniquet. This produces whole arm analgesia rather than blockade of individual nerves.
- Tourniquet is deflated after 20 min.

Epidural anaesthesia
- In this technique local anaesthetic (bupivacaine with or without diamorphine) is injected into the extradural space of the spinal cord via a thin catheter. It then diffuses through the nerve sheaths into the CSF.
- A great advantage of epidural anaesthesia is that the catheter can be left in situ, thus enabling continuous infusion of local anaesthetic.
- Epidural anaesthesia causes sympathetic nerve blockade in the region of infiltration, leading to vasodilatation and hence hypotension. This can be corrected with IV fluids and/or sympathomimetic drugs (e.g. ephedrine).

Spinal anaesthesia
- In this technique local anaesthetic (bupivacaine) is injected directly into the CSF in the spinal cord. The onset of action is

therefore faster than with epidural anaesthesia and a smaller dose is needed to achieve the desired effect.
• Spinal anaesthesia wears off after 3–4 h.
• Spinal anaesthesia causes sympathetic nerve blockade in the region of infiltration, leading to vasodilatation and hence hypotension. This can be corrected with IV fluids and/or sympathomimetic drugs (e.g. ephedrine).

Atracurium

Class: Non-depolarising muscle relaxant

Indications
- To achieve muscle relaxation in general anaesthesia
- Mechanical ventilation in ITU

Mechanism of action
- Atracurium competitively binds to nicotinic acetylcholine receptors at motor end-plates, antagonising the neurotransmitting action of acetylcholine. This causes paralysis of skeletal muscle. One major result is immediate loss of spontaneous respiration.

Adverse effects
- *Common*: rash, flushing, hypotension
- *Rare*: anaphylactoid reaction, bronchospasm

Contraindications
- Hypersensitivity

Interactions
- *Aminoglycosides*: these enhance the effects of atracurium
- *Botulinum toxin*: atracurium enhances neuromuscular blockade
- *Clindamycin*: this enhances the effects of atracurium

Route of administration
- IV

Note
- Non-depolarising muscle relaxants of short/intermediate duration of action (e.g. atracurium, vecuronium) are more widely used than those of long duration of action (e.g. pancuronium). Atracurium has an intermediate duration of action (30–45 min), and its onset of action is within 1–3 min. Duration of action is prolonged in hypothermia and myasthenia gravis.
- Non-depolarising muscle relaxants are not thought to cause malignant hyperpyrexia. They have no analgesic or sedative properties.
- Atracurium must only be used by experienced clinicians with facilities to support ventilation.
- The action of atracurium is reversible with an anticholinesterase agent (neostigmine).
- Atracurium is unique as it undergoes inactivation in the plasma and thus can be used in patients with hepatic or renal impairment.

Related drugs
- Cisatracurium, mivacurium, pancuronium, rocuronium, vecuronium

Isoflurane

Class: Inhalational general anaesthetic

Indications
- Maintenance of anaesthesia

Mechanism of action
- Exact mechanism is not fully understood.
- Most theories infer that general anaesthetic agents act on the cell membrane.
- Three important theories have been put forward:
  1 Lipid theory – anaesthetics change the lipid component of cell membranes and thus alter transmembrane ion movements to produce anaesthesia.
  2 Protein theory – anaesthetics bind to proteins and reversibly change their structure to induce anaesthesia.
  3 Hydrate theory – anaesthetics produce crystals within cell membranes by freezing the water component of the membrane, thus producing anaesthesia.

Adverse effects
- *Common*: coughing and breath-holding on induction due to pungent odour (hence not used for induction), respiratory depression, hypotension, tachycardia
- *Rare*: hepatotoxicity

Contraindications
- Hypersensitivity
- Malignant hyperpyrexia

Interactions
- *Antihypertensives*: these enhance the hypotensive effect of isoflurane
- *Epinephrine*: risk of possible cardiac dysrhythmias if given with epinephrine
- *Muscle relaxants*: isoflurane potentiates the effects of muscle relaxants

Route of administration
- Inhalation (via anaesthetic machine)

Note
- Volatile liquid anaesthetics (such as isoflurane) require carrier gas for administration. Nitrous oxide/oxygen mixtures, air and oxygen are all used for this purpose.
- Isoflurane is used in preference to halothane and enflurane as it has a much lower incidence of hepatotoxicity.
- Isoflurane has little effect on cardiac output or blood pressure, unlike halothane and enflurane.

Related drugs
- Desflurane, enflurane, halothane, sevoflurane

Lidocaine (lignocaine)

Class: Local anaesthetic, class I antiarrhythmic agent

Indications
- Local anaesthesia
- Ventricular dysrhythmias (especially following MI)

Mechanism of action
- Lidocaine blocks fast sodium channels in nerve axons. This leads to the following:
  1 Inhibition of generation of action potentials, thus causing a reversible nerve conduction block.
  2 Suppression of premature ventricular beats and ventricular tachycardia by slowing the conduction velocity along the Purkinje fibres and ventricular muscle in the heart.

Adverse effects
- *Common*: nausea, vomiting, drowsiness, dizziness, perioral tingling (all are signs of toxicity)
- *Rare*: CVS toxicity: bradycardia, hypotension, cardiac arrest; CNS toxicity: convulsions, confusion, coma

Contraindications
- IV administration is contraindicated in the following:
  - All degrees of AV node block and SA node disorders
  - Myocardial depression/severe cardiac failure
  - Porphyria

Interactions
- *Beta blockers*: these increase the risk of myocardial depression

Route of administration
- IV (dysrhythmias only); subdural, epidural; intradermal or subcutaneous injection at a desired site; topical application to mucous membranes and skin

Note
- Extreme care must be taken to avoid accidental IV injection during administration of local anaesthesia.
- Duration of local anaesthesia is prolonged when lidocaine is administered with epinephrine (due to local vasoconstriction).
- Solutions containing lidocaine and epinephrine must not be used in ring block anaesthesia (e.g. fingers, toes, penis) as this may cause ischaemic necrosis. Instead, solutions containing only lidocaine should be used.
- Lidocaine should not be injected into inflamed or infected tissue as this may cause systemic effects (due to rapid absorption from these sites).

Related drugs
- Bupivacaine, prilocaine, ropivacaine (all are purely local anaesthetics)

Neostigmine

Class: Anticholinesterase

Indications
- Reversal of non-depolarising muscle relaxants
- Myasthenia gravis

Mechanism of action
- Neostigmine inhibits the enzyme acetylcholinesterase in the synaptic cleft of neuromuscular junctions. This leads to a build-up of acetylcholine in the synaptic cleft and causes the desired cholinergic effects of enhanced neurotransmission.

Adverse effects
- *Common*: abdominal cramps, hypersalivation, diarrhoea (all due to excessive muscarinic effects)

Contraindications
- Intestinal obstruction
- Urinary obstruction

Interactions
- *Aminoglycosides*: these antagonise the effects of neostigmine
- *Clindamycin*: this antagonises the effects of neostigmine
- *Lithium*: this antagonises the effects of neostigmine

Route of administration
- Oral, IM or subcutaneous (all for myasthenia gravis); IV (for reversal of non-depolarising muscle relaxants)

Note
- Neostigmine has a short duration of action (2–4 h).
- Adverse effects of neostigmine can be counteracted by an antimuscarinic agent (e.g. atropine or glycopyrronium).
- Signs of overdose include bronchoconstriction, increased bronchial secretions, involuntary defecation, excessive sweating and nystagmus.
- Neostigmine does not cross the blood–brain barrier and hence has negligible central effects.
- Neuromuscular transmission may be impaired if excessive doses of neostigmine are given. This may lead to cholinergic crisis, which may be indistinguishable from worsening myasthenia gravis.

Related drugs
- Distigmine, edrophonium, pyridostigmine

Nitrous oxide

Class: Inhalational agent

Indications
- Maintenance of anaesthesia (in combination with inhalational anaesthetic agents)
- Analgesia without loss of consciousness (e.g. in labour)

Mechanism of action
- Exact mechanism is not fully understood.
- Nitrous oxide may act through inhibition of both NMDA glutamate receptors and non-NMDA glutamate receptors in the CNS.

Adverse effects
- *Rare*: bone marrow suppression, megaloblastic anaemia (both following prolonged exposure)

Contraindications
- Pneumothorax (air pockets in closed spaces may expand)
- Bowel obstruction

Interactions
- *Methotrexate*: nitrous oxide increases the antifolate effect of methotrexate

Route of administration
- Inhalation

Note
- For analgesia during labour, nitrous oxide is used as a mixture of 50% oxygen and 50% nitrous oxide. This can be employed as patient controlled analgesia.
- Nitrous oxide is not effective enough to be used on its own in surgery. However, it is widely used as a carrier gas for general anaesthesia in combination with other agents (e.g. isoflurane).
- Low blood solubility of nitrous oxide leads to rapid induction and recovery. Nitrous oxide has little effect on the cardiovascular or respiratory systems.

Propofol

Class: Intravenous anaesthetic agent

Indications
- Induction of anaesthesia
- Total intravenous anaesthesia
- Sedation during diagnostic and surgical procedures
- Sedation in intensive care

Mechanism of action
- Exact mechanism is not fully understood.
- There is evidence to suggest that propofol may act at $GABA_A$ receptors in the CNS.

Adverse effects
- *Common*: bradycardia, apnoea, hypotension, pain on injection
- *Rare*: anaphylaxis, convulsions, pulmonary oedema

Contraindications
- None

Interactions
- *ACE inhibitors*: these enhance the hypotensive effect of propofol
- *Beta blockers*: these enhance the hypotensive effect of propofol
- *Calcium channel blockers*: these enhance the hypotensive effect of propofol
- *Neuroleptics*: these enhance the hypotensive effects of propofol

Route of administration
- IV

Note
- Propofol is widely used due to rapid recovery rate without nausea and 'hangover' effect.
- Slow administration is recommended in the elderly and hypertensive patients, as a marked decrease in blood pressure can occur with rapid administration.
- Propofol induces sleep in one arm–brain circulation time (3–5 s).
- The pain caused by IV injection can be reduced by infiltrating lidocaine into the injection site prior to administration.

POISONING AND OVERDOSE

AIMS OF TREATMENT
• Decrease absorption of the substance (perform gastric lavage or whole bowel irrigation, or give activated charcoal)
• Increase elimination of the substance (e.g. by forced alkaline diuresis or haemodialysis or haemoperfusion)
• Give specific antidote where appropriate

GENERAL MANAGEMENT
• Resuscitate the patient (**A**irway, **B**reathing, **C**irculation)
• Make every attempt to obtain a history (what, when, how much and route of exposure)
• Physical examination may give clues to substance taken (e.g respiratory depression –opiates, benzodiazepines)
• If the substance is known, follow specific management as shown below
• If the substance is not known, blood and urine samples should be taken for toxicology screen and 4-hourly paracetamol and salicylate levels should be taken
• If specialist advice is needed, call the appropriate national or regional poison centre
• Provide supportive treatment
• Treat any complications (e.g. dysrhythmias hypoxia, hypotension, convulsions, hypothermia)
• If overdose was intentional, the patient should undergo a psychiatric assessment once recovered

Management of some common specific overdoses/poisons

ASPIRIN
- Measure plasma salicylate levels and plot on nomogram to guide treatment
- Perform gastric lavage (aspirin can delay gastric emptying, so lavage can be beneficial even hours after overdose)
- Give activated charcoal
- Replace fluid and electrolyte losses
- In severe overdose consider IV sodium bicarbonate (to achieve forced alkaline diuresis) or haemodialysis

PARACETAMOL
- Perform gastric lavage if within 1 h of ingestion and give activated charcoal if < 8 h since ingestion
- Measure plasma paracetamol levels (if at least 4 h have elapsed since ingestion) and plot on nomogram
- If levels are in toxic range, give IV *N*-acetylcysteine infusion (if within 24 h of ingestion) or alternatively give oral methionine (if within 10–12 h of ingestion).
- Monitor LFTs, INR, U&Es and ABGs
- If there is continued deterioration (i.e. encephalopathy, rising INR, renal failure, metabolic acidosis), contact local liver unit as liver transplant may need to be considered

TRICYCLIC ANTIDEPRESSANTS
- Give activated charcoal 4-hourly until clinical condition improves
- Attach cardiac monitor and monitor acid–base status and ventilation
- Treat any associated complications (e.g. convulsions, cardiac dysrhythmias)
- Acidosis should be corrected with sodium bicarbonate
- Dysrhythmias usually settle with correction of hypoxia and acidosis

BENZODIAZEPINES
- Supportive therapy usually suffices
- Flumazenil (a benzodiazepine antagonist) is only indicated for rare, life-threatening overdoses, i.e. respiratory depression or respiratory arrest

OPIATES
- Give IV or IM naloxone (a short-acting opioid antagonist), which can be repeated until breathing is adequate
- Due to the short half-life of naloxone, patients should be observed after administration

IRON
- Perform gastric lavage if within 1 h of ingestion or if X-rays reveal tablets in the stomach
- Give IV or IM desferrioxamine (an iron-chelating agent) depending on serum iron levels and clinical state
- In severe iron overdose not responding to chelation therapy, haemodialysis is indicated

DIGOXIN
- Perform gastric lavage if within 4 h of ingestion
- Give activated charcoal
- Correct any potassium disturbance and treat dysrhythmias with antiarrhythmic drugs (i.e. amiodarone, lidocaine)
- Give digoxin-specific antibody in serious overdose
- If digoxin-specific antibody not available, provide supportive treatment for dysrhythmias using a combination of antiarrhythmic drugs, overdrive pacing and D.C. shock

LITHIUM
- Increase fluid intake orally or IV to increase urine production and elimination of drug
- Provide supportive treatment
- Sometimes whole bowel irrigation is considered to decrease absorption of lithium
- In serious overdose perform haemodialysis

CARBON MONOXIDE
- Give 100% oxygen
- Measure carboxyhaemoglobin levels
- Consider giving hyperbaric oxygen if carboxyhaemoglobin levels > 20%, patient is pregnant, neurological symptoms are present or cardiac dysrhythmias occur

CYANIDE
- Give IV dicobalt edetate followed by IV dextrose

BETA BLOCKERS

- Give IV atropine for hypotension and cardiac dysrhythmias
- If this fails, give IV glucagon (to achieve a positive inotropic effect)
- Sometimes temporary pacing may be required if above measures fail

THEOPHYLLINE

- Perform gastric lavage (only within 2 h of ingestion)
- Give repeated activated charcoal 4-hourly until clinical condition improves or until charcoal appears in faeces
- Correct any hypokalaemia with IV potassium chloride
- Cardiac monitoring is required (as there is a danger of cardiac dysrhythmias)
- Give IV diazepam for any associated convulsions
- *Note*: tachycardia, hyperglycaemia and hypokalaemia may be reversed with IV propranolol (contraindicated in asthmatics)

ORGANOPHOSPHATES (insecticides, nerve gases)

- Wash contaminated skin and remove soiled clothing
- Give atropine (IV or IM) to antagonise the effects of acetylcholine which are intensified by organophosphates
- Pralidoxime mesilate can be used as adjunct treatment (further reduces the effects of acetylcholine)

This chapter is aimed to help with memorising lists of drugs that are frequently asked about in pharmacology exams. For some lists we have given more than one mnemonic – choose whichever suits your memory better!

HEPATIC ENZYME INDUCERS
GP Parcs
- Griseofulvin
- Phenytoin
- Phenobarbitone
- Alcohol (chronic use)
- Rifampicin
- Carbamazepine
- Sulphonylureas

HEPATIC ENZYME INHIBITORS
sickfaces.com
- Sodium valproate
- Isoniazid
- Cimetidine
- Ketoconazole
- Fluconazole
- Alcohol (in binge drinking)
- Chloramphenicol
- Erythromicin
- Sulphonamides
- Ciprofloxacin
- Omeprazole
- Metronidazole

PRODRUGS
CFC McZeal/Camelz CCF
- Carbimazole
- Fosphenytoin
- Cyclophosphamide
- Methyldopa
- Cefuroxime axetil
- Zidovudine
- Enalapril
- Azathioprine
- L-dopa

ZERO ORDER KINETICS
Pasta
- Phenytoin
- Alcohol

- Sodium valproate
- Theophylline
- Aspirin (only in high doses)

DRUGS METABOLISED BY ACETYLATION
Shippd/pH dips
- Sulfasalazine
- Hydralazine
- Isoniazid
- Procainamide
- Phenelzine
- Dapsone

DRUGS THAT UNDERGO EXTENSIVE HEPATIC FIRST-PASS METABOLISM
Soviet KGB lamp
- Salbutamol
- Opioids
- Verapamil
- Isoniazid
- Ergotamine
- Tricyclic antidepressants
- Ketoconazole
- Glyceryl trinitrate
- Budesonide
- L-dopa
- Antipsychotics
- Morphine
- Propranolol

RENALLY EXCRETED DRUGS
FHM balm ads/Sad Lamb FHM/Lambs Ham FD
- Fibrates
- Histamine 2 antagonists:
  - Cimetidine
  - Ranitidine
- Metformin
- Beta blockers (water-soluble):
  - Atenolol
  - Nadolol
  - Sotalol
- Antibiotics:
  - Aminoglycosides
  - Cephalosporins
  - Penicillins
  - Tetracycline

- Trimethoprim
- Vancomycin
- Lithium
- Methotrexate
- Azathioprine
- Digoxin
- Sulphonamides

DRUGS EXTENSIVELY BOUND TO PROTEINS
PDF swamp
- Propranolol
- Diazepam
- Fibrates
- Sulphonylureas
- Warfarin
- Aspirin
- Montelukast
- Phenytoin

DRUGS CAUSING HEPATITIS
I'm sharp scampi
- Isoniazid
- Methyldopa
- Sulphonylureas
- Halothane
- Amiodarone
- Rifampicin
- Phenytoin
- Sodium valproate
- Ciprofloxacin
- Antifungals (systemic)
  - Fluconazole
  - Ketoconazole
- Methotrexate
- Pyrazinamide
- Isotretinoin

DRUGS CAUSING PHOTOSENSITIVITY
PC start lag
- Psoralens
- Ciprofloxacin
- Sulphonylureas
- Thiazides
- Antipsychotics
- Retinoids
- Tetracyclines
- Loop diuretics
- Amiodarone
- Griseofulvin

DRUGS CAUSING LUPUS
Pig's pH
- Propylthiouracil
- Isoniazid
- Griseofulvin
- Sulphonamides
- Phenytoin
- Hydralazine

DRUGS CAUSING WEIGHT GAIN
Ms Clot
- Monoamine-oxidase inhibitors
- Sodium valproate
- Corticosteroids
- Lithium
- Oral contraceptives
- Tricyclic antidepressants

DRUGS CAUSING GYNAECOMASTIA
Madman's CK cog
- Metoclopramide
- Amitriptyline
- Digoxin
- Methyldopa
- Alkylating agents
- Neuroleptics
- Spironolactone
- Cimetidine
- Ketoconazole
- Cyproterone
- Oestrogens
- Gonadotrophins

DRUGS CAUSING PERIPHERAL NEUROPATHY
VIP scan
- Vinca alkaloids
- Isoniazid
- Phenytoin
- Sulfasalazine
- Cisplatin
- Amiodarone
- Nitrofurantoin

DRUGS CAUSING PULMONARY FIBROSIS
Bad Breathlessness Makes More Air Necessary
- Busulfan
- Bleomycin
- Methysergide
- Methotrexate
- Amiodarone
- Nitrofurantoin

DRUGS CAUSING PANCREATITIS
Fast cats
- Furosemide
- Azathioprine
- Sodium valproate
- Tetracycline
- Corticosteroids
- Alcohol
- Thiazides
- Sulphonamides

DRUGS CAUSING PROLONGED QT INTERVAL
QT tapes
- *Note*: Many drugs may cause prolongation of QT interval.
Some important examples are shown below.
- Quinidine
- Terfenadine
- Tricyclic antidepressants
- Amiodarone
- Phenothiazines
- Erythromicin (IV administration)
- Sotalol

DRUGS CASING GUM HYPERTROPHY
Community Psychiatric Nurse
- Ciclospirin
- Phenytoin
- Nifedipine

Index